The Diet Myth

Keeping Your Heart

Forever Young

The Diet Myth
Keeping Your Heart
Forever Young

Richard M. Fleming,
M.D., F.I.C.A., F.A.C.A., A.S.N.C.
Preventive Cardiologist
The Center For Clinical
Cardiology & Research

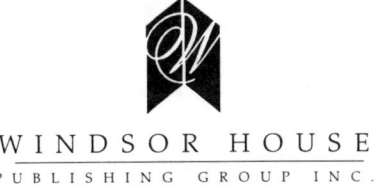

WINDSOR HOUSE
PUBLISHING GROUP INC.

Windsor House Publishing Group
Austin, Texas

THE DIET MYTH
KEEPING YOUR HEART
FOREVER YOUNG

Copyright © 1998 Richard M. Fleming M.D.
All rights reserved.

Written by Richard Fleming, M.D., F.I.C.A., A.S.N.C.

Edited by Ann C. Lang

Reproduction in any manner, in whole or in part,
in English or any other language, including usage of electronic,
mechanical, information storage or retrieval systems, or
any systems developed in the future, without the express
written permission from the publisher and author, except by a reviewer,
under the Fair Usage Doctrine, is strictly prohibited.
Any unauthorized use of any of the contents of this book
may result in civil penalty or criminal prosecution.
This copyright is registered with the U.S. Copyright Office,
Washington, D.C., and is protected under copyright law, and
internationally with all member countries of U.S./foreign copyright treaties.

PRINTING HISTORY
First Edition November, 1998

ISBN: 1-881636-70-4
Library of Congress Card Number: 98-061621

Windsor House Publishing Group, Inc.,
11901 Hobby Horse Court, Suite 1516
Austin, Texas 78758

The Windsor House logo is a trademark belonging to
The Windsor House Publishing Group, Inc.

PRINTED IN THE UNITED STATES OF AMERICA
10 9 8 7 6 5 4 3 2 1

Table of Contents

Chapter One.
The American Diet. 1

Chapter Two.
Diet Trends, Diet Fads, Pills and Surgery. 8

Chapter Three.
Is the Food We're Eating Killing Us? 23

Chapter Four.
The Truth about Food Labeling and the Food Pyramid. 47

Chapter Five.
The Vegetarian Myth, the Role of *Stress*, Blood Types, Your Horoscope and Hormones for Sale. 57

Chapter Six.
What's all the Confusion about Cholesterol? 66

Chapter Seven.
What's Causing Heart Disease and Strokes? 75

Chapter Eight.
Common Sense About Losing Weight. .85

Chapter Nine.
One Thing About Fast food, *It's Fast*. .91

Chapter Ten.
Improve your diet and enjoy what you're eating. 113

Chapter Eleven.
Healthy Happy Holiday Eating. 122

Chapter Twelve.
If We Don't Change the Direction We're Going,
We Will End Up Where We're Headed. 162

Chapter Thirteen.
Concluding Thoughts. 171

Introduction

In 1910 when the United States was relatively rural, most people worked hard (physically) and ate relatively little saturated fat. The amount of cholesterol they ate was about the same as we eat today, yet they didn't die from heart disease, cancer, high blood pressure or diabetes like we do today. They also weren't as overweight as we are. Today heart disease is the number one killer of both men and women and 25-35 percent of all children between kindergarten and twelfth grade have high cholesterol levels, diabetes, are overweight or have high blood pressure.

Americans and Europeans alike have been obsessed with their weight and having an ideal figure, while at the same time eat more calories and saturated fat than ever before. Since most of us no longer work on farms, but live in cities, we have been fascinated with health clubs and resorts in an effort to shed those extra pounds. In spite of all this, people continue to gain weight (an average of 7-10 pounds each Christmas/holiday season) and have more health problems than ever before. The diet industry has profited from all this by selling millions of dollars of remedies to consumers and they want you to believe that their product will take care of all your problems. The diet craze began as early as the 1890s and continues today. People who are desperately trying to lose weight and become healthier are searching for the fountain of youth in every diet that comes along. They assume if it's written it must be true. All too often they diet (which assumes no permanent change in eating habits, just something you do until you grow tired of it) and then return to their old eating habits, gaining even more weight than they originally lost, and the lifelong yo-yo diet begins.

Much of the information written today has no research or basis of support except for what the authors claim they have which has never been proven in the scientific community. These are in fact "feel good books." Too often however it is the author that feels good and not the person reading the book. In 1997 I published *How to Bypass Your Bypass: What Your Doctor Doesn't Tell You About Cholesterol and Your Diet*. This is one of only two books based on research published in the medical literature. Unlike the other book, this one is based upon 13 years of research and it continues to be valid because it is sound, practical, and continues to work long after the novelty has worn off. If you're a women you may not become a 36-24-26, and if you're a man you're probably not going to become the perfect inverted triangle, but the picture of perfect health and what is true health are not usually the same thing. If you're interested in the truth about many diets, then read on. If not, then put this book back on the shelf until you're ready for THE TRUTH.

Chapter One.
The American Diet.

Today we are inundated with television and radio ads telling us how to lose weight rapidly and fit into the clothes we want to wear. Books line the shelves of book stores telling us what we want to hear; that the book you're looking at will help you get the body you want where every other book has failed. **This book** is not based on a miracle cure or a gimmick. It is not based upon a few patients seen in the office or "a good idea." It is based upon many medical studies that we have published and presented in both the United States and Europe. Our original book *How to Bypass Your Bypass: What Your Doctor Doesn't Tell You About Cholesterol and Your Diet* discussed some of the earlier information you need to know to reduce your risk of heart disease, strokes, cancer, diabetes, high blood pressure and how to lose weight and keep it off.

> **THIS BOOK IS BASED UPON THE RESULTS OF MEDICAL RESEARCH – NOT A GIMMICK OR MIRACLE CURE.**

In this book we're going to look at the myths used to confuse people about health and diets. The key to all of these lie in starting with an idea that is true or seems like it should be true and then to lead you through a series of ideas in a way that makes you think you're agreeing with the author. The author may then tell you that he/she has seen people benefit from their approach. There is no published medical study to support most of the claims made by the author(s), but since the author is typically a doctor, nurse, pharmacist, dietitian or nutritionist, you assume they must be right and that they wouldn't mislead you. So with trust you accept their conclusions. It also helps to have a celebrity endorse the book. We trust our celebrities even though they have no expertise in the area. Being on a diet doesn't make you an expert, or most of us would be one.

> **JUST BECAUSE THE BOOK IS WRITTEN BY A SUPPOSED EXPERT – DOESN'T MEAN IT'S TRUE.**

Eating disorders affect many people with most of us convinced that we must do something about what we're eating. Most people don't know what to do and therefore we follow one diet after another. High protein, low carbohydrate and/or low fat/no fat diets are the most popular. In 1890-1900 most people thought the more you weighed the healthier you were. The reason for this was obvious at the time. In 1900 most people didn't have enough to eat, so if you were overweight you must have had a lot of money (to buy food) and if you had a lot of money you must also be healthier, or so people thought. So being overweight equaled health. The same problem happens today when people come from poorer backgrounds and make more money than their parents. As a result, many of these people who grew up with less, have ended up hurting themselves because of poor eating habits and dietary indulgences that their parents could not afford.

> **IN 1900 BEING OVERWEIGHT WAS HEALTHY. IN 1930 BEING THIN WAS HEALTHY. HEALTH ISN'T THE SIZE OF CLOTHES YOU FIT INTO.**

By the 1920s-1930s many more people became affluent and clothing styles changed. The "flapper" era lead to this new society seeking a slimmer image and a slimmer figure was then considered healthier. There was no more evidence to support this idea, than the heavier is healthy approach of twenty years earlier or the dietary myths of today. The number one cause of death among adults before the discovery of antibiotics was infection (eg. pneumonia), not heart disease, strokes, obesity, cancer, high blood pressure, or even diabetes. In 1928 Sir Alexander Fleming discovered the antibiotic penicillin and fewer people died from such infections, allowing us the opportunity to live longer, healthier lives.

> **THE DISCOVERY OF ANTIBIOTICS IMPROVED THE QUALITY OF OUR LIVES.**

With the arrival of the "great depression" getting enough food became a problem again and overeating was less of a problem. The second World War began in 1939 and preservation of food improved. This lead to the hydrogenation of food. This process of "saturating fats" helps to extend the shelf life of packaged (boxed) foods. Unfortunately this also tends to be the food we reach for most of the time. In 1910 an average person ate 166 pounds of saturated fat, by 1972 an average person ate 710 pounds of saturated fat in their lifetime. There are almost 3 million calories in saturated fat.

> **AN AVERAGE AMERICAN CAN EAT 3 MILLION CALORIES IN SATURATED FAT IN THEIR LIFETIME.**

By 1960, Americans and Europeans had fewer deaths from infection (thanks to the appropriate use of antibiotics), had more leisure time, were less physically active (now trying to replace the physical labor of their parents and grandparents with "workouts"), and were eating more "saturated fats." The amount of cholesterol in the diet hadn't significantly changed. Despite better medical care and fad diets, people started to die from obesity, heart disease, strokes, diabetes, and high blood pressure at ever increasing rates. By 1998, one million Americans are dying yearly from heart disease, 4000 a day, one every 20 seconds, with one-third to one-half having no idea they have a problem until they die from a heart attack. In addition, one person will experience a stroke every minute and every four minutes someone will die from a stroke-related problem.

> **1 MILLION AMERICANS DIE EACH YEAR FROM HEART DISEASE. 4000 EVERY DAY. ONE EVERY 20 SECONDS.**

Despite much debate about cholesterol and triglycerides (fats in the blood), when the level of cholesterol and triglycerides are greater than 150 (mg/dl), the risk of dying from heart disease and cancer increases dramatically. Conventional tests (coronary angiograms/catheterization) see only the larger arteries and miss the small and medium sized blood vessels where the effect of early disease can be most pronounced. One of our patients, a 32-year-old lady with a cholesterol level of 178 and chest pain which got worse with exercise, was seen elsewhere before coming to participate in our program. The angiogram of the arteries of her heart showed no disease, and she was told she had no heart problems. This test (angiogram), which many people have to look for heart disease, places a tube into an artery in the groin or arm. Another tube is placed inside it and advanced into the arteries of the heart where a contrast agent (typically referred to as dye) is injected and x-rays are taken.

> **ONE AMERICAN WILL HAVE A STROKE EVERY MINUTE. EVERY FOUR MINUTES A PERSON WILL DIE FROM A STROKE-RELATED PROBLEM.**

Because of her persistent chest pain, we did a Positron Emission Tomography (PET) study to more accurately look at both the blood flow to her heart and to determine if her heart had suffered any damage prior to her coming to see us. The results are shown in figure 1 (page 5) where each picture represents the heart with the tip of the

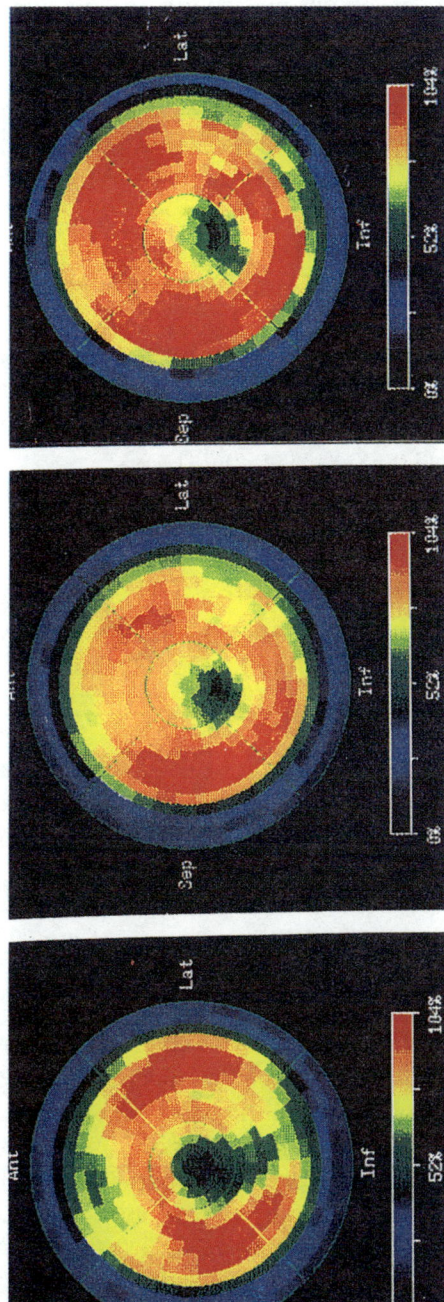

Figure 1

heart at the center of the image. The top of the image represents the top part of her heart while the bottom of the image represents the bottom of her heart. The three o'clock and nine o'clock positions represent two other walls of her heart. Good blood flow is shown as red, with yellow representing less blood flow, and blue depicting even less. When she first saw us, the image to the far left represented the maximum blood flow her heart was receiving. The top, tip (middle) and bottom of her heart had "severe" disease. The center picture shows her after six months with improvement after following our recommendations and the last image (far right) shows further improvement yet after 18 months of treatment. The tip of her heart failed to show improvement and other studies we did showed she had already had a heart attack in this area of her heart without knowing it, and she was only 32 years old.

> **IF YOUR CHOLESTEROL OR TRIGLYCERIDES (FAT) ARE GREATER THAN 150, THEY'RE PROBABLY ALREADY TOO HIGH.**

The basis for reversing her heart disease is laid out in the lifestyle changes discussed in *How to Bypass Your Bypass: What Your Doctor Doesn't Tell You About Cholesterol and Your Diet*. It is not a diet or extremism approach which you abandon over time, but a reasonable lifestyle change that **you can live with**. It begins with determining the number of calories you need (figure 2). If you weigh 150 pounds, you need 1500 calories a day. Of these 1500 calories, 15% should be protein (not necessarily meat, but it doesn't exclude meat either) and 15% should be fat — but not "saturated fat" which is usually found in meats and dairy products. This means that eating meats and dairy products with little or no "saturated fat" isn't a problem, unless you're eating too many calories. Fifteen percent of 1500 calories is 225 calories in protein and fat as shown in figure 2. Since protein has 4 calories per gram, you will need (225 calories/ 4 calories per gram) 56 grams of protein. More than adequate for most people.

Figure 2. Balancing your caloric needs.

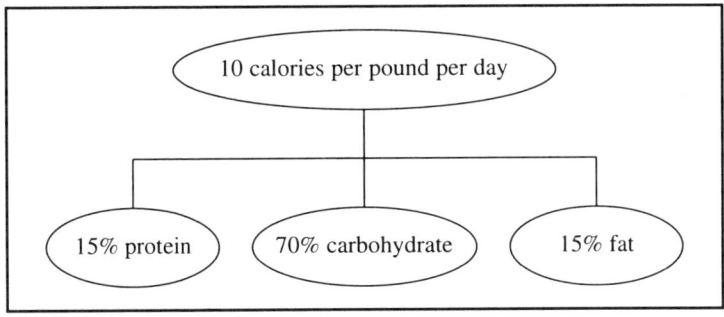

Since fat has 9 calories per gram you will need (225 calories/ 9 calories per gram) 25 grams of fat to help maintain your body's health. People who develop diabetes when they become adults do so in many cases because they are eating too many calories. These extra calories can come from sugar, but they can come from any source (fats, protein, or carbohydrates) and are not limited to unhealthy foods. With our approach you start with the number of calories needed (10 calories per pound per day) to determine the right number of calories for the day. For our hypothetical 150 pound person, 70% of the 1500 calories a day comes to 1050 calories. Since there are 4 calories per gram of carbohydrate, this means that the person needs (1050 calories/4 calories per gram) 262 grams of carbohydrates daily to maintain their weight of 150 pounds.

In the next chapter, we're going to look at many of the dietary trends/fads over the last 100 years and how they could be hurting both you and your family.

Chapter Two.
Diet Trends, Diet Fads, Pills and Surgery.

The definition of a "diet" according to the *American Heritage Dictionary* of the English Language is: "The usual food and drink of a person or animal; daily sustenance." "A regulated selection of foods, or especially as prescribed by a doctor for gaining or losing weight or for other medical reasons." "Anything taken or provided regularly." Unfortunately, a "diet" according to most people is something they "go on" to lose weight and then look forward to "going off."

> **MOST AMERICANS THINK A DIET IS SOMETHING YOU GO ON TO LOSE WEIGHT & THEN GO OFF (AND REGAIN THE WEIGHT).**

In the 23rd edition of *Stedman's Medical Dictionary*, diet is defined as "Food and drink in general." The medical dictionary then goes on to define not one, not two or even three diets, but 41 different types of diets; not a one of which is named after someone living today. The confusion about dieting is not new and popular diets used today include "high-protein," "low-protein," "high-carbohydrate," "low-carbohydrate," "high-fat," "low-fat," 'high-calorie' and 'low-calorie' diets." In other words, everything from one extreme to the other. Most other diets, regardless of their names, reflect one of these diets or a theme associated with them. In this chapter we're going to review some of the popular diets used over the last 100 years and examine some of the problems seen with them.

RICHARD M. FLEMING, M.D.

> **TODAY'S DIET FADS RANGE FROM ONE EXTREME TO THE OTHER, WITH YOU CAUGHT IN THE MIDDLE.**

While diets probably date back to antiquity, the modern American diet has experienced a number of trends which get renamed (the names are changed to protect the not-so innocent) depending upon who is promoting them. For example, diets which emphasize eating fewer foods with carbohydrates include the Atkins diet, the Zone (books 1 and 2), the sugar buster theory and the Scarsdale diet. All of these diets emphasize that carbohydrates result in elevated insulin levels and you will potentially end up with all the problems seen with diabetes. The truth behind these arguments is that if you're someone who developed diabetes later in life, you probably have higher insulin levels than someone who didn't develop Adult Onset Diabetes Mellitus (AODM).

> **IF HIGH CHOLESTEROL LEVELS ARE DUE TO HIGH INSULIN LEVELS, THEN WHY DO MOST PEOPLE WITH HIGH CHOLESTEROL HAVE NORMAL INSULIN LEVELS?**

Many of these authors suggest that higher cholesterol levels in these individuals are due to an elevation in insulin levels and that too many calories are being eaten as carbohydrates – which includes not only sugar, but other sugars, complex carbohydrates like starches and dietary fiber which everyone knows you need. However, if high insulin levels were the cause of heart disease and elevated cholesterol levels, it doesn't explain why the majority of people with high cholesterol levels do not have diabetes. Some of these books also say that flaxseed oil lowers cholesterol levels. However we know this is not true, because published medical research has shown that it is the solid part of the flaxseed that lowers cholesterol levels, not the oil. More importantly is that the books stating that the flaxseed oil lowered cholesterol were published before any research was done to determine whether the oil lowered the cholesterol level or not. This is not only an example of something published without proof, but the use of a popular idea everyone wanted to believe in so badly that the truth (an idea was good enough) didn't seem to be as important as the idea the authors wanted to promote.

> **THE SOLID PART OF FLAXSEED LOWERS CHOLESTEROL, NOT THE OIL.**

As early as the 1890s some people suggested they knew how to lose weight. No proof, they "just knew." One of these earliest ideas proposed that if you chewed your food 100 times before swallowing it, this would improve your digestion of food and you would lose weight. I remember growing up as a boy with my parents telling me to chew my food thoroughly. I also remember them telling us that chewing each bite of food 100 times would improve the digestion of the food. This was in the 1960s and the idea had persisted for more than fifty years. While I don't suggest to my children that they eat their food whole (I don't like the idea of them choking), I also know there's no benefit behind chewing each bite of food 100 times. The benefit behind such an approach probably laid in the fact that people became more aware of their being "full" because of the amount of time it took to eat. It might have also been due to fatigue or just plain boredom from all the chewing. If this method were truly the best way to lose weight, then the use of food processors should have shown a tremendous drop in our level of obesity, since you can really pulverized food in a food processor. This early approach to compulsive chewing may very well have been the first "liquid diet."

From 1915-1920 people began to count calories; however, little if any information followed to suggest if the life-long counting of calories provided the desired effect. Little if any information regarding protein, carbohydrate or fat intake was included in these dietary programs. During this time, people became very interested in how much they weighed and the first bathroom scales were produced.

While the dietary approach may have left little impact, the sale of bathroom scales has soared. Good news if you made bathroom scales. During the 1930s women (who smoked very little, primarily due to social taboos) were encouraged to smoke cigarettes rather than eat. The phrase "reach for a Lucky instead of a sweet" was a popular advertisement. Unfortunately, this habit of cigarette smoking (exchanging one bad habit for another) would gain popularity and later be shown to have adverse health risks.

> **WE HAVE CONFUSED HEALTH WITH APPEARANCE.**

By the 1930s women discovered that if they couldn't lose it, they could cover it up, hiding those mid-life bulges with the "latex girdle." While this didn't make them weigh less, they "looked" better. Diet fads began to gain ground and the notorious grapefruit diet/Hollywood diet was born. People on this diet ate grapefruit (which like oranges have a natural appetite suppressant), green leafy vegetables, melba toast (which you can still find) and hard-boiled eggs. While the eggs provided the only true protein source (not to mention cholesterol) on this diet, the emphasis wasn't placed on balance, but reducing the total number of calories you ate, and probably wanted to eat after being on this diet for a while. This was the truly first "diet" as most people use the term today. People only went on this "diet" for 18 (this must have seemed like a good number or maybe it's all people could tolerate) days. After the 18 days they were on their own again. Since people ate an average of less than 700 calories a day on this diet, they were guaranteed to lose weight, not to mention protein (muscle), water and maybe their mind. Diets which result in more than 1-2 pounds of weight loss per week may not only be dangerous, but frequently accomplish this weight loss by muscle and water loss (dehydration).

> **YOU SHOULD TRY TO LOSE ONLY ONE TO TWO POUNDS PER WEEK – MORE COULD BE HARMFUL.**

THE DIET MYTH

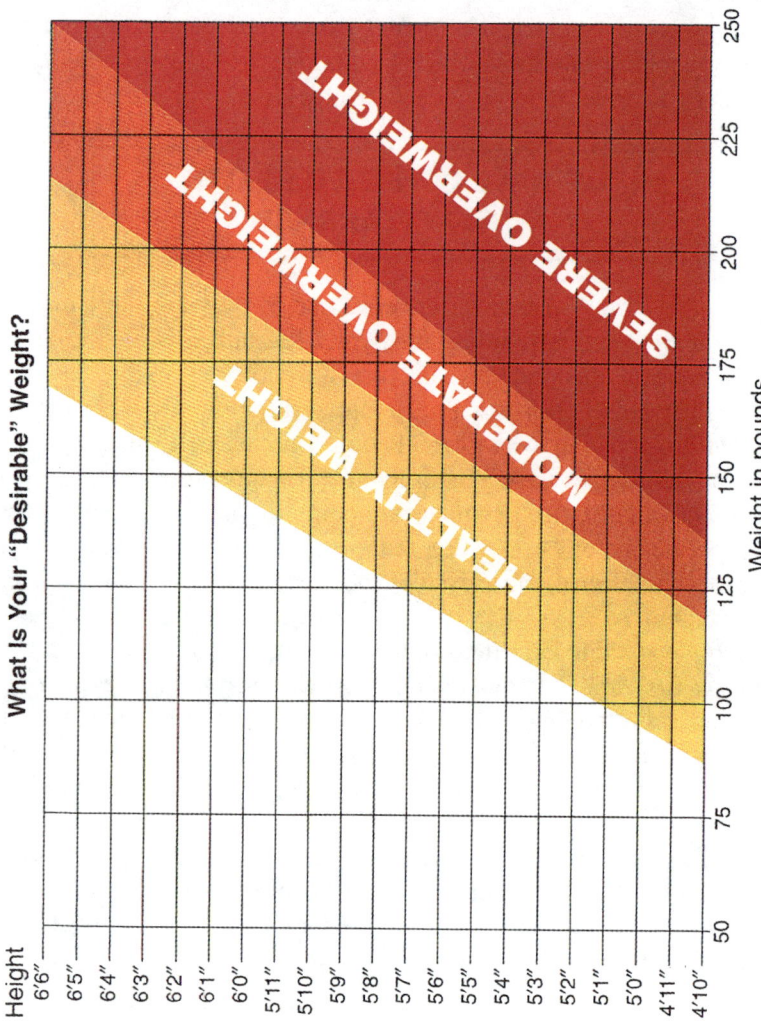

Figure 1

By the 1940s information about life expectancy based upon height and weight began to be published and used for life-insurance purposes. A good example of a height and weight scale is shown in figure 1. While the weights on these tables have continually been shifted upward, primarily because people are getting heavier and heavier, little of any attention was focused on the increased death rate seen in people who were and are underweight. Such an emphasis has been placed on being overweight, that anorexic individuals still see themselves as overweight, despite looking like prisoners of war. In fact many (but not all) contestants of beauty pageants have been known to induce vomiting to help them lose weight and remain competitive. Women are not the only ones who place themselves at increased risk by "purging" themselves. Men have followed suit, particularly in the athletic arena (e.g. wrestlers) where athletes who are trying to reach a certain weight for competition will starve themselves to get to a lower weight class.

During the 1940s prescription medicines began to emerge as a medical treatment for obesity. The idea being that if you couldn't lose weight by reducing the amount of food you ate, you could increase the metabolism of your body and subsequently lose weight as long as you remained on the "pills." The use of these stimulant medications, which without a prescription would be the equivalent of "speed/uppers" (illegal street drugs), also lead to increased heart rate, blood pressure, and the potential for heart attacks and strokes. In fact, while I practiced in Houston, Texas, men and women who were admitted to the hospital for heart attacks who where in their 20s and 30s were routinely checked for amphetamine (eg. crack cocaine) use.

Figure 2. The balance between calorie intake and calorie needs.

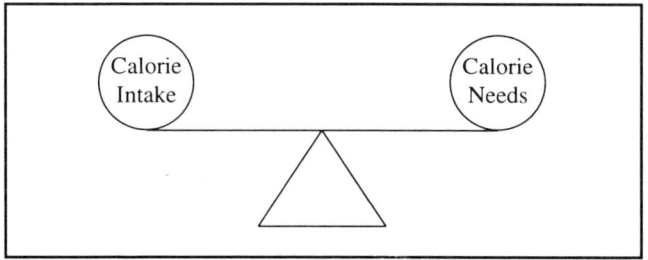

During the last 50 years, studies looking to lower cholesterol levels included the use of thyroid hormone. This was based upon the "observation" that people with lower than normal thyroid levels had higher cholesterol levels. This is a classic example of someone's observation of a problem without research to support it. The studies which were conducted using thyroid hormone to lower cholesterol levels in people with normal thyroids, showed an increase in the number of deaths among these people, and today this approach is considered unacceptable. There's a world of difference between an idea and reality.

> **THERE'S A WORLD OF DIFFERENCE BETWEEN A GOOD IDEA AND REALITY.**

Despite information like this, the search for a "magic pill" which will allow people to lose weight without changing their eating habits continues. Just this year (1998) the combination of fenfluramine and phentermine (fen-phen) was stopped by the Food and Drug Administration (FDA) because of damage seen on the valves of the heart in people taking these two prescription medications. The fen-phen combination was supposed to be used only for people who were severely overweight, although I have seen such patients with damaged heart valves who clearly did not meet the weight qualifications, yet many of them received the drugs anyway. While some people may have escaped damage, many others did not, even though many of them took the drugs for "short" periods of time.

Despite the shock to the American public, herbal remedies were rapidly promoted to try to take the place of the popular fen-phen combination. These were described as "herbal fen-phen" and promised weight lose without side-effects. The message should have been clear, you don't put something in your mouth to treat something you've already put in, you simply don't put the first thing in your mouth. It doesn't matter whether it's a prescription drug, an "herbal remedy," a laxative or cathartic.

> **YOU DON'T TREAT SOMETHING YOU PUT IN YOUR MOUTH BY PUTTING SOMETHING ELSE IN, YOU TREAT IT BY NOT PUTTING THE FIRST THING IN!**

Another dietary method has been to try to "trick" your body by eating "virtual" sugar and fat substitutes which either have no caloric value or are not absorbed by your body. This began with Saccharin in 1958, and was followed by NutraSweet in 1982 and Olestra in 1998. While there are many concerns surrounding these artificial ("virtual") foods (e.g. cancer and/or the loss of fat-soluble vitamins like Vitamins A, K, E and D), the market for low-calorie low-fat substitutes continues. I call these "Virtual-Calories," because like "Virtual-Reality," they are not "real."

> **VIRTUAL CALORIES HAVE NO NUTRITIONAL VALUE.**

In addition to "Virtual-Calories" a number of companies have developed foods designed to appeal to your interest in losing weight. While some of these may be helpful, many are focused on key words which you (as the consumer) assume have a different meaning. For example, "reduced fat" milk may be reduced, but not that much. "Reduced fat" milk is really 2% milk which has been relabeled, based upon the interest of consumers to buy low-fat foods. However, 2% milk means that 35.7% of the calories are fat calories. Not what I really consider "reduced fat."

Another example is "No-fat margarine." There is nothing illegal about calling your margarine "No-fat margarine," because it's just a name and the food label shows us that 100% of the calories are fat calories. A manufacturer can call their product just about anything they want to, "caveat emptor" (let the buyer beware), it's up to you to sort out the truth. Finally (for now), one of my favorite examples is the advertisement that different brands of peanut butter have no cholesterol. The reality is that no peanut butter has cholesterol, unless it is artificially added to it. The average 2 tablespoon serving (probably less than most people use) of regular peanut butter has no cholesterol, but more than 70% of the calories are fat calories.

> **YOU CAN CALL A FOOD ABOUT ANYTHING YOU WANT TO, AS LONG AS THE FOOD LABEL IS RIGHT – SO READ THE FOOD LABEL.**

As I mentioned in the first chapter, our parents and grandparents lived more physically challenging lives, which in part accounted for their ability to use up most of the calories they ate. Since then we have tried to find ways to increase the number of calories that we use up in a day, without changing the amount of food we're eating. This has led to an entire industry with so-called experts willing to sell or promote a product which will flatten your "tummy," "hips," and build those muscles you're looking for. We have more work-out videos, exercise equipment, and health instructors available to use than a Roman Gladiator.

Our exercise craze was popularized by Jack LaLanne and his television program in the 1950s and 60s. Others have followed with workout videos, exercise clubs/studios and infomercials galore. While I encourage exercise (exercise is a good thing), you have to do a lot more exercising than you think to use up the number of calories you want. Not to mention having a misguided motive behind the exercise which will eventually result in more frustration and discontinuation of the exercise program and its benefits. The first book, *How to Bypass Your Bypass* talked about the number of calories you use for activities ranging from sleeping (0.43 calories per pound per hour) to walking (4.22 calories per pound per hour) at 5.3 mph. This means that if you weigh 150 pounds, you will use up 64.5 calories each hour you sleep and 633 calories each hour you walk at 5.3 mph, assuming you can keep up this pace for one hour.

> **EXERCISE IS GOOD BUT DON'T DO IT SO YOU CAN HAVE ANOTHER COOKIE.**

People tend to focus on what they can eat as a result of their "workout" instead of the benefits derived from the exercise itself. If you're interested in losing weight, one of the best exercises you can do is to push yourself away from the table. If you're interested in an exercise program try walking for 30 minutes, three to five times a week, taking the stairs instead of the elevator or parking farther from the store and walking. This not only is good for you but your children, grandchildren or others who are important in your life. If you're trying to achieve your maximum ("target" heart rate) desirable heart rate, this is determined by your age as shown in figure 2. Subtract your age from 220. Take 70% of this number and that is the heart rate you should try not to exceed. Some people should try not to exceed 50% depending upon other health problems. As usual you should be checked by a physician before starting on an exercise program to make certain it is safe to do so.

Figure 2. Determining Your Target Heart Rate.

Target Heart Rate = (220 - age) x (0.70)

By the early 1970s a number of diets were backed by physicians and others with impressive credentials. In fact, the more impressive the better. You've undoubtedly heard the expression "If you can't dazzle them with brilliance, baffle them with ..." – you know the saying. These credentials suggest a scientific basis, but the approaches were not backed up by scientifically published medical data and we've already seen with the thyroid treatment study how dangerous this approach can be.

The most common of these diets are the "high-protein," "low-carbohydrate" diets. The idea being that eating too many carbohydrates causes increased insulin levels. These diets have **multiple side-effects** including ketosis (excessive acid production by the body), calcium loss (from your bones) with potential osteoporosis, kidney damage and elevations in cholesterol levels. The reality is, if you do not provide your body with enough carbohydrates from which to make glucose (sugar) to run your body (particularly your brain) your liver will make the sugar it needs (gluconeogenesis) from the proteins (muscles) in your body. Regardless of the name given to these diets, they can have serious consequences. Fortunately, most people don't stay on diets long enough to suffer the full impact of these diets or we would probably see even more problems.

> **IF YOU DON'T GIVE YOUR BODY GLUCOSE (SUGAR) IT WILL MAKE IT FROM THE MUSCLES OF YOUR BODY.**

Another variant of these "Virtual-Diets," so named because they are diets you cannot stay on for extended periods of time, include the low-fat diets. The problem, as we and others have published in both the medical and lay journals, is that "saturated fat," not "fat" in general, is the culprit which we must be concerned with. The main problem with meat in the diet is the amount of "saturated fat" found in most meats. This is why the preparation of food is so important. For example, if you grill meat and let the fats drip out of the meat, then there is less of the saturated fat remaining for you to eat. However, if you fry the meat or let it sit in the fat after cooking, the meat will reabsorb all the "saturated" fats and you will then eat them, which will subsequently increase your cholesterol and triglyceride (fat) levels.

> **IT'S NOT THE MEAT BUT THE SATURATED FAT IN THE MEAT THAT PRODUCES THE PROBLEM.**

Despite the bad reputation it has received, fat is a necessary component of a healthy diet and we need 7.5 grams of linoleic acid daily if we are to fight of infections and make the membranes for each of the cells of our body. This polyunsaturated (Linoleic Acid) fat is essential to our health and can be found in vegetable oils including safflower, sunflower, corn and soybean oils. To obtain this amount of linoleic acid, we need a diet with at least 10% fat, but preferably 15%. Diets which eliminate fat altogether can therefore produce significant health problems. The Pritikin diet for example promotes a high-fiber diet but reduces fat consumption to less than 10% as does the Ornish Diet and the Beverly Hills Diet. The Beverly Hills Diet emphasizes nothing but fruit for six weeks. This is a diet which clearly isn't intended to last forever and therefore won't be of benefit long-term because you return to other eating habits after the six weeks are over. While you're on it, however, you can be guaranteed regular bowel movements. In fact, diarrhea is a common problem.

> **"LOW-FAT" DIETS LIMIT OUR ABILITY TO FIGHT INFECTION AND MAKE THE CELLS OF OUR BODY. IT'S THE SATURATED FATS WE NEED TO REDUCE, NOT ALL FATS.**

Other diets like the one popularized by Dean Ornish emphasizes reducing the daily fat intake to less than 10% of your total calories and becoming vegetarian. This approach assumes that meat and all fat are the primary problems with the American Diet, and ignores the issue of excess calories. This is only partially correct in that it is the excess in "saturated fat" (either from excess calories or directly from saturated fat itself) and not the meat itself which is the problem. Coincidentally, one of the major problems with this approach is the failure to control the number of calories eaten. Many people on this diet increase the number of calories they eat to compensate for what they view as a stringent diet, only to find out that these excessive calories (from non-meat sources), like all excess calories (regardless of the source), get turned into fat. You don't have to graduate from medical school, you probably don't even have to graduate from high school to know that if you eat more calories than you need, the calories get stored as fat. These excess calories, stored as fat, drive up the triglyceride (fat) levels, which then drive up the cholesterol levels and increase the risk of heart disease.

THE DIET MYTH

> **IT'S NOT WHAT YOU'RE EATING, BUT WHAT'S IN WHAT YOU'RE EATING THAT'S IMPORTANT.**

The answer (while I'm 98-99% vegetarian myself) isn't the elimination of all meat or fat from the diet, but reducing the "saturated" fat and controlling the overall number of calories eaten, so good calories are not stored in the body as fat calories. Recently I attended a talk by someone promoting a number of soy products. This person has written a number of books about vitamin therapy and was promoting more vitamins, minerals and soy products through a company he was involved with. These products were conveniently available for purchase right there at the talk. During the talk, samples were given out of a 1.7 ounce soy bar which had 186 calories, of which 36 were fat calories. This means that this reportedly "nutritious" "super energy bar" had almost 20% of its calories coming from fat, and one-half of these were "saturated" or "bad" fats. Looked at from another perspective, 5 ounces of this soy bar had about the same amount of fat as a 5 ounce sirloin steak. Interestingly enough the idea was that this soy bar was better for you because it was made out of soy and everyone knows soy is better for you than the steak, RIGHT?

> **EVEN SOMETHING THAT SOUNDS LIKE IT'S GOOD FOR YOU CAN BE BAD FOR YOU IF IT'S FILLED WITH GARBAGE.**

Some diets like the Mediterranean and Hawaiian diet have higher levels of fat than we have in the mainland United States or Europe. The difference lies in the type of fat eaten. The Mediterranean and Hawaiian diets can easily be 40% fat. Most of the fat is polyunsaturated fat. The other important point is that these people do not eat more calories than they need and therefore do not have excess calories to turn into fat. The Tarahumaran Indians, typically used to demonstrate how heart healthy eating results in little if any heart disease, were studied after being feed diets similar to most Americans. As a result the Tarahumaran Indians showed an increase in their weights, cholesterol levels and glucose levels in as little as 5 weeks. The Tarahumarans returned to normal once they returned to their traditional way of eating.

> **THE TARAHUMARAN INDIANS SHOWED AN INCREASE IN WEIGHT, CHOLESTEROL AND GLUCOSE LEVELS FIVE WEEKS AFTER EATING AN AMERICAN DIET.**

Notwithstanding the plethora of diets, pills, exercise programs, gimmicks, and infomercials, modern medical science has come to the aid of those who can not or will not control their appetite. With the addition of Liposuction and other cosmetic surgeries, the general public's image of a healthy/beautiful body can be maintained artificially if not naturally. Yes, you can have the figure you want assuming you have the money to pay for it and you're willing to accept the potential risks involved. Of course, this won't change your eating habits, but you can always have more surgery. In essence, we have returned to the 1890-1900 era, where with enough money you can buy the picture of health, even if it's not health itself. The external appearance is what too many of us look at.

> **THERE'S A DIFFERENCE BETWEEN EXTERNAL BEAUTY AND INTERNAL HEALTH.**

In 1998 more than 1 million Americans will die from heart disease, and much of what causes heart disease nutritionally can also be linked to strokes, diabetes, high blood pressure and some cancers. This dietary/nutritional trend is even worse for younger individuals. Today 25 to 35% of our children between kindergarten and twelfth grade have high cholesterol, high blood pressure, diabetes or are overweight. In fact when the National Lung and Blood Institute conducted a study in 1996, they discovered that 40% of all nine- and ten-year-olds were trying to lose weight. Despite this, 35% of the calories children are eating are fat calories (regardless of age, sex, race or family income) due to poor dietary habits, which we're teaching them at school and at home. In addition, they are spending less time engaged in vigorous physical activities and more time being sedentary; problems which have lead to our health problems and are increasing our childrens' health problems.

For the last 23 years I have been involved with the American Heart Association in one manner or another; including talking, researching, and writing on the subject of heart disease for the last 13 years. During this time the dietary habits of the majority of Americans and Europeans have not improved much, and for many have gotten worse. In the next chapter we are going to look at how the American diet has lead to increases in heart disease, strokes, high blood pressure, diabetes and weight problems.

Chapter Three.
Is the Food We're Eating Killing Us?

The human body needs six nutritional elements to survive: protein, carbohydrate, fat, vitamins, minerals and water. The elimination of any one of these will eventually lead to death. The overconsumption of any of these will lead to health problems and eventually death. Many people, recognizing that we will all die someday, have adopted the attitude of "who cares." You're going to die of something and it might as well be something you enjoy. A movie I once saw sums up my feelings on this approach very well, "many things can kill you, but you'd be surprised what you can live through." For all too many people, illness and not death is the result of poor dietary and lifestyle practices. In this chapter we will discuss how our six nutritional elements can have an effect on cancer, heart disease, high blood pressure, obesity and diabetes mellitus. You are after all, what you eat.

<u>HOW MUCH FAT IS TOO MUCH</u>
&
<u>HOW LITTLE IS TOO LITTLE</u>

Fat, despite all the misrepresentation of it in popular books, the news and medical literature, is a necessary component of our life. Many people think about fat in terms of where it comes from (or where we have it on our body) versus what type it is and the effect it has on our bodies. The fat we eat, regardless of where it comes from, is one of three types: "saturated," "monosaturated" and "polyunsaturated." Saturation refers to the chemical appearance of the fat as shown in figure 1. The more <u>hydrogen</u> atoms you add to something the more <u>hydrogenated</u> it becomes. Hydrogenation and saturated are different terms for the same process. The more saturated a food is, the longer it will last on the shelf and probably in you. Saturated fats are the ones that lead to increases in your blood cholesterol and the subsequent buildup of cholesterol in the arteries of your body, including your heart and neck.

Figure 1. Saturated, monosaturated or polyunsaturated.

Saturated Fatty Acid	$H-\underset{H}{\overset{H}{C}}-\underset{H}{\overset{H}{C}}-\underset{H}{\overset{H}{C}}-\underset{H}{\overset{H}{C}}-H$
Monosaturated Fatty Acid	$H-\underset{H}{\overset{H}{C}}-\underset{H}{C}=\underset{H}{C}-\underset{H}{\overset{H}{C}}-H$
Polyunsaturated Fatty Acid	$H-\underset{H}{C}=\underset{H}{C}-\underset{H}{C}=\underset{H}{C}-H$

C = carbon, H = hydrogen

The average American eats 58 grams of "saturated" fat each day. The total fat eaten daily has increased from 125 grams per person per day in 1910, to 168 grams per person per day today. This represents a 35% increase in total fat calories. In fact, the greatest percentage of the calories we eat are coming from fat, which now makes up more than 40% of our daily calories. One might think that our children, eating in our public schools, would be eating healthier than we are. Unfortunately 38% of the calories our children eat are fat calories. As table 1 shows us, the greatest percentage of our fat is coming from meat and this fat is primarily "saturated."

Table 1. Principle Sources of Today's Dietary Fats.

Source of Fat Calories	Percentage of Total Fat Calories
Meat, fish, poultry	41%
Milk and milk products	17%
Grain products	15%
Fats & Oils	10%

When we look at the trends over the past 20 years, the major increase in fat eaten by us is due to the processing (hydrogenation/saturation) of foods and the use of salad and cooking oils. As a result more and more Americans are plagued with obesity and 30% of all school-age children are overweight.

> **OUR CHILDREN ARE EATING ALMOST 40% OF THEIR CALORIES IN FAT.**

This excess of fat in our diet has lead to an explosion of weight problems, heart disease, strokes and cancer. There is a positive relationship (correlation) between dietary saturated fat consumed and these health problems. As the amount of fat in the diet increases there tends to be more bile acids released by the gallbladder to aid in the digestion of the additional fat. The increased production of bile acid and its release into the intestines has been associated with an increased risk of colon and rectal cancer. Part of this problem may lie in the fact that diets with more fat also tend to have less fiber. This reduction in fiber means there will be less stool and the result is a more concentrated bile, which may cause colon cancer.

> **MORE SATURATED FAT AND LESS FIBER CAN LEAD TO BOTH HEART DISEASE AND CANCER.**

Regardless of whether one is eating too much fat, or too many calories (figure 2), the body makes fat from the additional calories. This extra fat can result in hormonal changes, including the conversion of male hormone into female (estrogen) hormone. This explains why men who gain body fat with age can have an increase in female hormone resulting in the development of some breast tissue (gynecomastia), and why women are more prone to develop breast cancer with increased dietary fat intake.

FAT CAN INCREASE ESTROGEN LEVELS.

Figure 2. Too many calories become fat, regardless of the source.

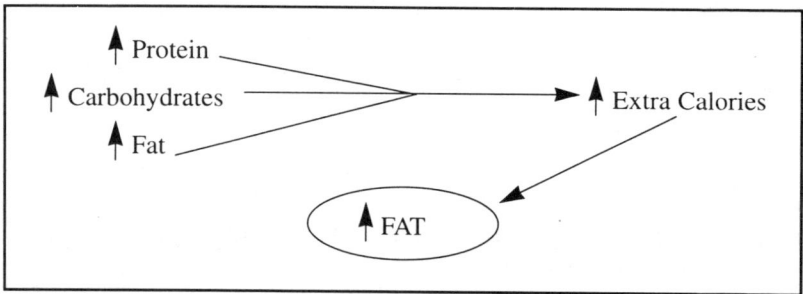

This excess fat made from extra calories results in the production of fats (triglycerides) which can supply up to two-thirds of the energy needed by the cells of our body. However, excessive triglyceride production can increase our cholesterol levels. These increased cholesterol and triglyceride levels lead to disease in the arteries of the heart and neck resulting in possible heart attacks and strokes. Not all fats (eg. polyunsaturated fats) have this effect, but when we eat too many calories, the fat produced increases our cholesterol levels. Assuming we are not eating too many calories, it is the "saturated" fats which will increase our cholesterol levels while the monosaturated fats have little or no effect. The polyunsaturated fats have been shown to actually decrease cholesterol levels. This explains why people who eat the right amount of calories, can eat higher amounts of polyunsaturated fat but have less heart disease than Americans and Europeans who eat more saturated fat.

> **TOO MANY CALORIES AND SATURATED FAT INCREASE CHOLESTEROL LEVELS, MONOSATURATED FATS HAVE LITTLE OR NO EFFECT ON CHOLESTEROL. POLYUNSATURATED FAT LOWERS CHOLESTEROL.**

So far we have discovered that too much fat, particularly "saturated" fat, can increase you risk of heart disease, strokes, weight problems and cancer. The obvious next question is whether it is possible to eat too little fat. The answer as you have probably guessed by now is YES! The polyunsaturated fat, Linoleic Acid, an omega-6 fatty acid, is found in safflower, sunflower, corn and soybean oils and is essential for life. It is therefore called an essential fatty acid (EFA). This EFA not only helps lower our cholesterol levels, but is necessary for the formation of every cell in our body. This outer part of each cell is called the "cell membrane" and it is partially composed of arachidonic acid which is made from Linoleic Acid. This is why cell function and integrity requires 7.5 grams of Linoleic Acid daily.

> **YOU NEED ABOUT 15% OF YOUR CALORIES IN FAT TO GET THE AMOUNT OF LINOLEIC ACID YOU NEED.**

Essential fatty acids are also needed for the production of chemicals in your body called prostaglandins, prostacyclins, interleukins, and thromboxane. These chemicals are responsible for regulating heart rate, blood pressure, blood vessel relaxation, blood clotting, nerve function and the absorption of carotene and vitamins A, K, E and D, without which we could not live. Diets which reduce fat intake to less than 10% of the total caloric intake places a person at risk of not getting adequate amounts of Linoleic Acid and should not be done without consulting your physician.

THE TRUTH ABOUT CARBOHYDRATES & WHY WE NEED THEM

A lot of emphasis has been placed on carbohydrates as the major cause of health problems in the United States and Europe. (The truth is it is too many calories and too much saturated fat.) Much of this focuses on the assumption that too much sugar is bad for you and makes children hyperactive and adults diabetic. The truth about hyperactivity in children and too much sugar is still being debated, but regardless of the outcome, it doesn't change the need for carbohydrates in our diet. While we could live without carbohydrates, diets which exclude them are potentially dangerous. Many people and books would lead you to believe that the entire problem is due to increased insulin levels caused by the carbohydrates we are eating. People who develop diabetes as they get older, and who are overweight, may have higher than normal insulin levels. The truth however is that most people do not have this problem despite eating more calories than they need and most people will not develop diabetes. It is also true that most people with high cholesterol levels have normal insulin levels.

> **MOST PEOPLE WITH HIGH CHOLESTEROL LEVELS HAVE NORMAL INSULIN LEVELS.**

All carbohydrates leave the small intestine (gut) as one of three sugars: glucose, fructose and galactose. These sugars are changed into glucose (in the liver) and then released into the blood for use by the body. With the aid of insulin (figure 3) the glucose enters the cells of your body where it is needed. As your blood sugar increases your insulin level goes up to help move the glucose into the cells of your body. Any extra calories get stored as glycogen and fat regardless of whether they begin as protein, carbohydrates or fat. Glycogen is sugar put together for use in the near future. Approximately 110 grams are stored in the liver and 225 grams in the muscles of your body. When people go on starvation diets (fasts), these stores are immediately used up, after which ketones (acids) may be produced as we will discuss below. Assuming you are not on some unusual diet, the average individual will have 10 grams of sugar (glucose) in the blood for immediate use by your body.

Figure 3. How insulin works in your body work.

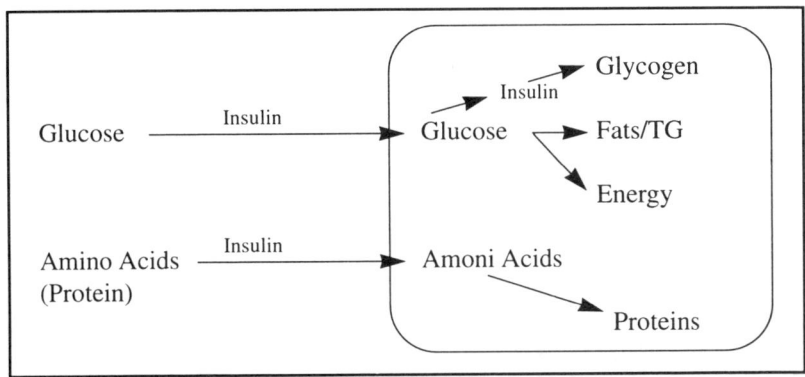

What people forget, or decide not to mention, when they promote high-protein, low-carbohydrate diets (with or without fat recommendations) is that insulin is necessary for protein as shown in figure 3. Insulin inhibits the breakdown of our muscle protein (gluconeogenesis). When we deprive our body of carbohydrates, we lower insulin levels and promote the breakdown of our muscles to make sugar for our body to run on.

Like fat, there is not just one type of carbohydrate, although many people would like you to think so. Carbohydrates consist of those which you can digest (break down and get into your body) and those you cannot. The latter is referred to as the total "dietary fiber" on food labels. These are the fibrous parts of plants including hemi-celluloses, celluloses and lignin. It is the lignins of flaxseed which have been scientifically shown to reduce cholesterol levels, and not the flaxseed oil, which so many popular books would suggest.

> **FLAXSEED OIL DOESN'T SIGNIFICANTLY EFFECT CHOLESTEROL, THE SOLID PART OF FLAXSEED IS WHAT WORKS.**

The digestible carbohydrates include sugars (glucose, fructose and galactose), dextrins (derived from starches) and starches (the plant equivalent of human glycogen). Regardless of what they begin as, all carbohydrates will be turned into glucose for use by the body. Table 2 shows the makeup of several common sugars we eat.

Table 2. Common (double/two sugars together) sugars we eat.

Common Name	Chemical Name	Actually Sugars
Cane or Beet Sugar	Sucrose	Glucose & Fructose
Malt or Beer Sugar	Maltose	Glucose & Glucose
Milk Sugar	Lactose	Glucose & Galactose

While many people think that Americans and Europeans are eating more and more carbohydrates the reality is that people alive in 1910 actually ate 20% more carbohydrates than we do today, with 56% of their calories coming from carbohydrates. So if carbohydrates are going down in comparison to 1910, people in 1910 should have had more problems with insulin, if insulin is the real culprit as so many people and books (without research to back them) have claimed. Carbohydrates, as we discussed in *How to Bypass Your Bypass: What Your Doctor Doesn't Tell You About Cholesterol and Your Diet*, have only 4 calories per gram, where fat (and we're eating more saturated fat today) has 9 calories per gram. Essentially we have replaced the lower calorie carbohydrates with the higher calorie (saturated) fats.

> **IF THE AMOUNT OF CARBOHYDRATE WE EAT AND OUR INSULIN LEVELS ARE WHAT CAUSES OUR HEALTH PROBLEMS, OUR GRANDPARENTS WHO ATE MORE CARBOHYDRATES THAN WE DO SHOULD HAVE HAD MORE HEALTH PROBLEMS THAN WE DO!!!**

Today we eat an average of 408 grams of carbohydrates every day, which represents 46% of our total daily calorie intake. Approximately one-half of these come from starches with the other half (53%) coming from more refined sugars. In 1910 people ate an average of 492 grams of carbohydrates daily. The major difference is the types of carbohydrates we are eating. In 1910, 68% of the total carbohydrate calories were consumed as starches, with the other 32% coming from sugars. The overall trend has been a reduction in carbohydrates (replaced by saturated fats, which increase the total daily caloric intake) while at the same time decreasing the grains, breads, cereals and potatoes (starches) eaten, and increasing the consumption of sugars. This results in less fiber from the carbohydrates we do eat. Clearly, the problem isn't the amount of carbohydrates we're eating, but the types. This is the same problem we discovered when looking at fats in the diet; the major problem was the types of fats (saturated) eaten.

> **WE EAT FEWER CARBOHYDRATES THAN OUR GRANDPARENTS, BUT A GREATER % OF REFINED SUGARS.**

Finally let's look at what carbohydrates do for us. Carbohydrates (glucose) is the major source of energy used by our body. The brain (central nervous system) is so dependent upon it that failure to keep blood sugar levels in an acceptable range can result in a coma. When people substantially lower their consumption of carbohydrates, the body must turn to other sources for energy. This would be like using kerosene to run your car if you couldn't get gasoline. It might run for a while, but it wouldn't work very well. When this happens, your body starts to rip down the fat and protein in your body to make glucose. This is called gluconeogenesis (or the production of new glucose).

Your body is not designed to work this way except under adverse conditions and acids (ketones) are produced as a result. These acids combine with the sodium (salt) in your body and are excreted (removed from your body) in the urine. This additional loss of salt will remove water with it and result in dehydration (a great way to lose weight, but not very healthy on your body). In fact, this dehydration could result in blood pressure drops, decreased blood flow to the brain, brain damage, coma and possibly death (not good). There is also more uric acid produced as a result of the increased protein eaten, which frequently happens with these low-carbohydrate diets; subsequently gout and kidney damage can follow.

> **HIGH PROTEIN, LOW CARBOHYDRATE DIETS CAN CAUSE KIDNEY DAMAGE, DEHYDRATION, KETOSIS, MUSCLE DAMAGE, COMA AND OSTEOPOROSIS.**

Your liver is responsible for changing many of the toxic substances found in you into something which can be removed from your body. To do this your liver needs to make something called glucuronic acid, which it makes from glucose. This glucuronic acid combines with the toxic substances in your body, allowing them to be removed from you rather than continuing to accumulate and cause you harm. Additionally, carbohydrates which are indigestible remain in your colon and increase bulk to improve the removal of wastes (bowel movements) from your body. In doing so, it reduces the toxic effect of bile salts (and cancer) as discussed above. In fact, your body **needs** 20-35 grams of dietary fiber every day, including the soluble (dissolve in water) fibers found in legumes, vegetables and fruits with edible peelings (eg. pears and apples), and the insoluble fibers like cereals, wheat bran, whole-grain breads and cereals, and pastas. The definition of a legume (eg. dried beans and peas) is a food with the seeds inside of the pod. When the pod is split into its two halves or valves outlined by the seams, the seeds remain attached at the edge of one of the valves.

YOU NEED 20-35 GRAMS OF FIBER DAILY.

When carbohydrates are removed from the diet, particularly lactose (glucose and galactose) which remains in the gut longer than the other sugars, the growth of bacteria in our bowels is adversely effected. These bacteria need carbohydrates like lactose to grow. The bacteria are responsible for making vitamin K (which we need to help clot our blood) and many of the B-complex vitamins. The bacteria also help with the regularity of bowel movements.

The sources of carbohydrates in our diet are also very important sources of proteins (eg. grains and cereals), minerals and B-vitamins. Sugars obtained from the carbohydrates are also necessary for making nerves (galactosidases) and the tissue which helps hold our body together (connective tissues). Finally, the genetic codes of our body, deoxyribonucleic acid (DNA) and ribonucleic acid (RNA) require sugars to be made.

EVEN OUR GENETIC CODE HAS SUGARS IN IT.

THE DIFFERENCE BETWEEN ANIMAL ALANINE AND PLANT ALANINE

Protein, <u>all</u> protein, is made up of 20 different building blocks called amino acids. Regardless of where the protein comes from (animal, vegetable, grain, et cetera), the amino acid ALANINE looks the same, and every protein you eat (regardless of where it came from) is digested the same way. Proteins enter your mouth, they're chewed (at least by most of us) and then swallowed. Once in your stomach they are subjected to hydrochloric acid (HCL) and mixed like a food processor. (So technically, your stomach represents the first food processor.) Further enzymes released from your pancreas continue the process until the proteins are broken down into smaller proteins (peptides) or amino acids themselves.

> **THERE IS NO DIFFERENCE BETWEEN ANIMAL AND PLANT AMINO ACIDS.**

The digestion of food requires energy and much has been made of eating more protein and less carbohydrate and fat, to increase your metabolic rate. This increase in energy for the digestion of food is called the specific dynamic action (SDA) and is greater for protein than either carbohydrate or fat. This increase in energy need is not due to the actual digestion of food (as many think), but rather it is the heat produced by your liver breaking down this food. The SDA represents one-tenth of your basal metabolic rate (BMR). As we discussed in *How to Bypass Your Bypass*, the BMR averages 10 calories per pound per day. So if you're a 150 pound person, your BMR is 1500 calories per day. Put another way, you need 1500 calories each day to run your body. If you change what you're eating to include only protein (ignoring the damage caused to your body by doing so), you wouldn't increase your body's basic energy needs enough to justify eating another apple, which you couldn't do anyway since it's not in your diet. So much for the myth of changing what you eat to increase your body's metabolism.

> **YOU CAN'T CHANGE YOUR BODY'S METABOLISM ENOUGH BY CHANGING WHAT YOU EAT, TO JUSTIFY EATING DIFFERENTLY.**

Amino acids are looked at by your body in much the same way as fat is, there are those you need, and those you don't. Of the 20 amino acids your body needs, to build its own proteins, we can make all but 9 or 10 of these, depending upon how old you are. These 9 or 10 essential amino acids are listed in table 3 and are called essential (just like essential fatty acids), since they must be supplied to us in our diet for us to live.

> **OF THE 20 AMINO ACIDS WE CAN MAKE ALL BUT 9 OF THEM.**

Not all protein foods have all 9 or 10 of the essential amino acids we need. This is the basic difference between meat and non-meat sources of protein. Those foods which provide us with all the "essential amino acids" our bodies need are called **complete proteins** (eggs, milk, cheese and meats), whereas most plant proteins are missing at least one of the essential amino acids. This can be overcome by combining (figure 4) several **incomplete protein** sources together to make **"complementary proteins."** These are proteins which "complement" each other to provide us with all of the essential amino acids we need.

> **COMPLETE PROTEINS PROVIDE ALL OF THE ESSENTIAL AMINO ACIDS, WHILE COMPLEMENTARY PROTEINS MUST BE COMBINED TO GIVE THE SAME RESULTS.**

Examples of complementary proteins include milk and a wheat sandwich, beans and wheat, rice and beans, sesame seeds and rice, peanuts (peanut butter sandwich) and milk. The only thing which you need to remember is to combine these protein sources to get all the "essential" amino acids. Soy protein is the only known example of a "complete" vegetable protein. However, soybeans also have an enzyme (trypsin "inhibitor") which interferes with the digestion of its proteins. This "inhibitor" can be destroyed by simply cooking the soybeans, allowing the soy protein to become a "complete protein."

Table 3. The essential amino acids

The Twenty Amino Acids	Essential Amino Acids for Infants	Essential Amino Acids for Children and Adults
Arginine	Arginine	
Histidine	Histidine	Histidine
Isoleucine	Isoleucine	Isoleucine
Leucine	Leucine	Leucine
Threonine	Threonine	Threonine
Lysine	Lysine	Lysine
Methionine	Methionine	Methionine
Phenylalanine	Phenylalanine	Phenylalanine
Tryptophan	Tryptophan	Tryptophan
Valine	Valine	Valine
Alanine	not essential	not essential
Asparagine	not essential	not essential
Aspartic Acid	not essential	not essential
Cysteine	not essential	not essential
Glutamic Acid	not essential	not essential
Glutamine	not essential	not essential
Glycine	not essential	not essential
Proline	not essential	not essential
Serine	not essential	not essential
Tyrosine	not essential	not essential

Figure 4. Complementary proteins.

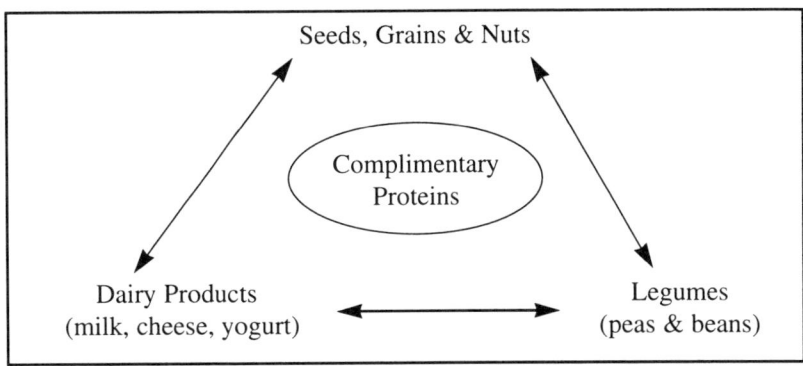

Infants (birth to 1 year) need roughly 1 mg of protein per pound per day. The protein requirements for children vary and are shown in table 4. The average adult needs 0.3-0.4 mg of protein per pound per day. Using the approach we outlined in chapter 1, figure 2, the person weighing 150 pounds would eat exactly the right amount of protein (56 grams of protein) they need in a day.

Table 4. Protein needs by age.

Age	Protein Needs
Infants (0-1 year)	up to 1 gram/pound/day
Children (1-3 years)	23 grams
Children (4-6 years)	30 grams
Children (7-10 years)	34 grams
Children (11-18 years)	45 grams
Adults years	0.3-0.4 grams/pound/day

As we mentioned earlier, the problem with the amount of meat in the diet, is not the fact that it is animal flesh, but rather the amount of "saturated" fat present in the meat. Many people talk about the amount of cholesterol in the meat and believe it is the cholesterol that is the problem. In reality, the cholesterol is in the lean part of the meat, while the "saturated" fats lie more in the "fat" or "marbled" part of the meat. In 3-1/2 ounces of untrimmed meat and 3-1/2 ounces of lean meat there would be little difference in the amount of cholesterol consumed, with the untrimmed meat having 94 mg of cholesterol and the trimmed meat having 91 mg. Put another way, equal amounts of fatty and lean meat have roughly equal amounts of cholesterol. So when we trim the fat off our meat we are reducing the saturated fat we would otherwise eat, not the cholesterol.

As we have already mentioned, the amount of cholesterol we eat has little effect upon the level of cholesterol in our blood, since the more cholesterol we eat, the less our liver typically makes, while increasing the amount of "saturated" fat we eat will increase the amount of cholesterol our liver makes.

Another major difference between vegetable and dairy proteins, versus meat proteins is the amount of ammonia the liver makes from the protein. More ammonia (which must be removed by the kidneys) is made from the animal proteins (SDA) than vegetable or dairy proteins. This is one of the reasons why people with kidney and liver disease must eat less protein than other people.

> **VEGETARIANS CAN ACQUIRE ADEQUATE AMOUNTS OF THE ESSENTIAL AMINO ACIDS BY USING COMPLEMENTARY PROTEINS.**

Clearly by balancing complementary proteins, vegetarians (and non-vegetarians) can obtain the necessary protein needed for optimal health. The purpose behind needing protein in our diet is to repair worn out body proteins, provide for growth of new tissue, and provide immunologic protection for the body. Since the beginning of the century there has been little change in the percentage of calories eaten daily as protein, despite what people might otherwise think. As outlined in table 5, changes in the American diet this century have primarily shown (significant) increases in (saturated) fat calories with concomitant reductions in carbohydrates, particularly the amount of starches eaten.

Table 5. Percent of daily calories consumed as fat, carbohydrate and protein in 1910 and today.

Year	% Fat Calories	% Carbohydrate Calories	% Protein Calories
1910	32	56	12
Today	43	46	11

WHAT IS A VEGETARIAN & ARE YOU ONE?

The term vegetarian has long been used to define people who do not eat meat, thereby depending upon complementary protein sources. There are at least 6 types of vegetarians who have different reasons for their dietary practices. Table 6 defines each of the various types of vegetarians. Regardless of philosophical differences, nutritional practices should be sound (as explained in this book) to reduce harm to the individual. There are many potential benefits to a vegetarian life-style, but there are also some potential problems as well. Major changes in nutritional practices should be done with discretion and guidance from qualified individuals and there are many people who would like you to believe that they are qualified to teach you how to reach perfection. The reality is that most of these people have questionable credentials and none of us have reached nervana.

Table 6. The six major types of vegetarians.

semi-vegetarian	eat dairy, eggs, chicken, fish, no other animal meat
pesco-vegetarian	eat dairy, eggs, fish, no chicken or other animal meat
lacto-ovo-vegetarian	eat dairy foods anad eggs, no other animal meat
ovo-vegetarian	eat eggs, but no dairy or other animal meat
vegan	no animal meat

As you can see the major differences reflect which (if any) meats, dairy products and/or eggs a person is willing to eat. Vegans need to be particularly concerned about getting enough vitamin B-12 (for nerve function) along with sufficient vitamin D and calcium (for bones). Vegans, like the ovo-vegetarians need to make sure they get adequate iron in their diets to reduce the risk of iron deficient anemia (IDA), which can be a particularly difficult problem if too much fiber or soy protein is eaten since both the fiber and soy may further reduce the amount of iron absorbed from the gut. Ovo-vegetarians, like vegans, can have problems not getting enough vitamin D and calcium, leading to increased bone loss with age (osteoporosis) or rickets in children.

> **THE SPECIAL NUTRITIONAL NEEDS OF VEGETARIANS CAN BE MET WITH A LITTLE PLANNING.**

If you decide to adopt a vegetarian lifestyle, there are certain foods you can eat to help improve your diet. Vitamin B-12 can easily be added by eating cereals and grains which have been fortified with B-12, in addition to soy milk. There are margarines fortified with vitamin D and additional vitamin D is made in your skin with exposure to sunlight; although the idea is not to develop skin cancer. Calcium can be found in many foods including tofu (soybean curd), kale, bok choy, legumes, green leafy vegetables, seeds, nuts, spinach (not a great source of iron as many think), collard greens, great northern beans, also grains and cereals when enriched with calcium. Iron can be added to the diet with green leafy vegetables, iron fortified grains and cereals, whole grains, dried fruits, tofu, and legumes. The amount of iron absorbed in the diet can be increased with vitamin C (which chemically reduces the iron, thereby increasing iron absorption in the small intestine). Vitamin C is found in citrus fruits and fruit juices, tomatoes, strawberries, black raspberries, broccoli, potato skins, peppers and dark green leafy vegetables.

RICHARD M. FLEMING, M.D.

THE BENEFITS OF CERTAIN VITAMINS AND MINERALS & HOW THEY COULD REDUCE YOUR RISK OF HEART DISEASE AND CANCER

A lot of attention has been paid recently to a group of vitamins and minerals called antioxidants. Substances called oxygen-free radicals (OFRs) are released as a result of chemical reactions in our body. These OFRs are extremely toxic and have been associated with certain types of cancer, heart disease, the aging process and potentially strokes. Vitamins and minerals which work within the body to prevent or limit the damage caused by OFRs are called antioxidants. These include vitamins C and E, beta-carotene (not vitamin A), selenium, and possibly others. A common medication used for heart patients (nitroglycerin) also works as an antioxidant. These vitamins are found in yellow-orange fruits, green-leafy vegetables and some fortified grains and cereals. Additional evidence suggests that some individuals may benefit from folate (folic acid) and B-complex vitamins – particularly B-6 and B-12.

We now know that the formation of OFRs produce further disease in the arteries of the heart (heart disease) and neck (leading to strokes) by at least three different methods. The <u>first</u> is an increased ability to deposit cholesterol into these arteries after the cholesterol has been made from "saturated" fats in our diet, or from extra calories we eat, regardless of whether they were protein, carbohydrates or fat. The <u>second</u> effect is to increase the amount of "oxidized" LDL cholesterol which causes further cholesterol buildup and arterial damage, and the <u>third</u> effect is to directly damage the blood vessels themselves. Homocysteine can aid in reversing these effects but requires adequate folic acid and vitamin B-12 in the diet to do so.

Apart from the effects on heart disease and stroke, several vitamins and minerals have been associated with reducing certain types of cancer. Selenium is a potential antioxidant which requires adequate soil levels if it is to be sufficiently present in the food we eat. If there are inadequate selenium soil levels, then the foods we eat will have insufficient selenium to be of much value to us.

Selenium deficiencies have been associated with colon and rectal cancer, as well as breast cancer. When iron is not adequately present in the diet, our immune system may be depressed and gastric cancer may increase. Not all problems are related to dietary deficiencies. There are some reports of too much zinc causing breast and stomach cancer. Too much or too little iodine is seen in some types of thyroid cancer.

> **VITAMINS C & E, FOLIC ACID, SELENIUM, IRON AND ZINC MAY ALL PLAY A ROLE IN PREVENTING CERTAIN TYPES OF CANCER.**

Vitamin C may not only reduce the risk of heart disease, it has also been shown that higher levels of vitamin C in the diet is associated with a lower incidence of gastric (stomach) and esophageal cancers. Vitamin C may do this by helping to build collagen which helps form a barrier to the cancer cells. Finally, Vitamin C and Vitamin E have been shown to inhibit the production of nitrosamines. Nitrosamines have been shown to cause certain types of cancer and are found in water and vegetables contaminated with some fertilizers or in "cured" meats. Vitamin E has also been shown to inhibit sarcomas (a type of cancer). Folic acid (folate) not only helps maintain our homocysteine levels in the fight against heart disease, but it can also help protect us against damage to our chromosomes/ genetic material.

The addition of artificial sweeteners has been an attempt to reduce the number of calories we're eating despite our failure to limit the amount of food we eat. Saccharin and cyclamate are two classic examples. Large doses of Saccharin has been shown to be associated with bladder and urinary tract cancers in rats, while toxic byproducts of cyclamate has been shown to cause chromosomal damage, testicular atrophy, skin damage (dermatitis) and convulsions in animals. Even the way in which we prepare our food, may not only lead to heart disease, but to cancer as well. Charcoal broiling, frying of foods and smoking of food has been associated with intestinal cancers as a result of polycyclic aromatic hydrocarbon (PAH) production which then permeates the food we are eating.

> **WHAT WE'RE ADDING TO OUR FOOD AND HOW WE'RE COOKING IT COULD BE KILLING US.**

Frequently it is impossible to determine the exact benefit any one vitamin or mineral can have against any particular type of cancer, because good dietary/nutritional habits not only include eating what's good for us, but avoiding that which is harmful. Animal studies have shown that eating too many calories can not only make animals diabetic, overweight and develop heart disease, but that these excess calories may be associated with cancer. Whether this is related to the effect of extra fat as discussed earlier in the chapter, or simply due to extra calories is not clear.

MAYBE I SHOULD JUST GIVE UP AND GO LIVE IN A CAVE SYNDROME

Well after reading the last section you may have decided to either go live in a cave somewhere or burn this book, or perhaps both. Before doing the latter two, read on. If after all the years I've spent researching heart disease and its reversibility I had come to the conclusion that all was lost, you wouldn't be reading this book right now because I wouldn't have been able to write it from the cave I would have gone to.

While there are a lot of things we can do to clean up the environment, the air we breath, the water we drink and the food we eat, it is impossible to return to the Garden of Eden. What we have learned is that we don't need to go to extremes to live longer healthier worth-while lives. We don't have to fast for weeks and purge our bodies of every toxin that ever entered them. We don't need to go on high-protein, low-carbohydrate diets that damage our bodies while we stay on them. We don't have to all become vegetarian or eliminate all the fat from our diet – nor should we. We also don't have to have the "perfect" body to be "perfectly" healthy. The purpose of this chapter was to point out many of the misconceptions in these extreme diets that people have been promoting (and will continue to

THE DIET MYTH

promote as long as the money's there) for the last 100 years, based upon peoples' fears and uncertainties. Feeding off these fears and uncertainties is like selling snake oil; they know it doesn't work, and you will too, but only after you've bought it.

> **THERE WILL ALWAYS BE PEOPLE WILLING TO SELL YOU SNAKE OIL AS LONG AS THERE ARE PEOPLE WILLING TO BUY IT.**

Healthy living and good nutrition is straightforward and relatively simple. It is based upon eating the right amount of calories, the right amount of protein, carbohydrate and fat for the amount of calories you should be eating. The change in the American and European diet during the last 100 years has been a shift away from sensible eating to one of extremism and convenience. While we have been increasing the amount of saturated fat in our diet, we have been decreasing the complex carbohydrates, which in the end are necessary for optimal health. Diets which promote further extremism aren't going to improve our health since we've already seen every extreme imaginable. The names of the diets keep changing to protect the not-so innocent.

Figure 5. A reasonable sound nutritional plan <u>you can live with</u>.

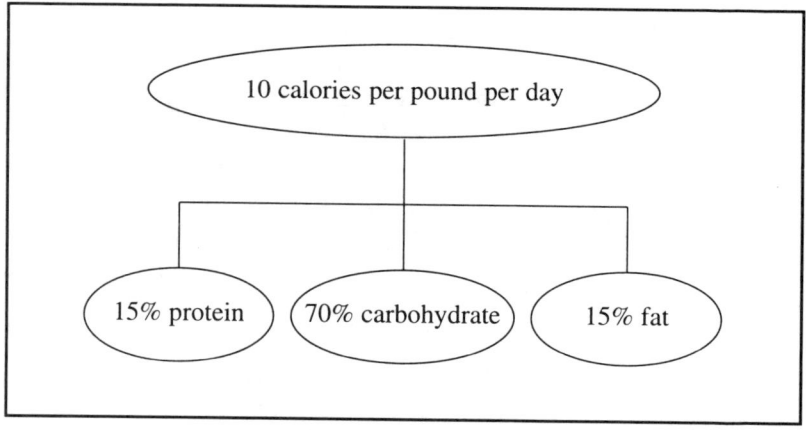

When dieters yo-yo from one diet to another they cause more potential health problems searching for the mythical figure of health and beauty, while getting the not so healthy results. Vitamins and minerals are important to help maintain the health of our bodies, but mega-vitamin schemes and infomercial specials don't provide a substitute for sound nutritional practices. Supplemental vitamins have no special benefit over the same vitamins found in our foods and there are no studies showing that extreme doses of each of these vitamins combined will protect you from heart disease, strokes, cancer or anything else. Sound nutritional advice suggests some potential benefits by increasing the recommended daily allowance (RDA) of some vitamins, but not to the extremes advocated by the people who are making a profit selling you these megadoses of vitamins and mineral supplements.

> **THERE ARE NO STUDIES TO SHOW THAT MEGADOSES OF MULTIPLE VITAMINS ARE GOOD FOR YOU.**

Table 7. Reasonable recommended doses of antioxidants vitamins

Vitamin	Daily Recommended Dose
Beta-carotene	5000 IU (international units) *
Folate	400 micrograms
Vitamin C	500 - 1000 milligrams
Vitamin E	100 - 250 (international units) *

* higher doses may have adverse side-effects

In addition to the above words of advice, we should eat more fruits, vegetables, and whole grain cereals and breads, eat less "saturated" fat, and avoid foods which are smoked, salt cured or pickled. Try to avoid foods which have nitrates added to them, stop smoking and drink alcohol in moderation. Keep your caloric intake to 10 calories per pound a day, with 15% of these calories coming from protein, 15% from fat (preferably polyunsaturated or monosaturated) and 70% from carbohydrates – remembering to eat more complex carbohydrates (2/3 of the carbohydrates) and fewer simple/refined (1/3 of the carbohydrates) carbohydrates.

Along with the above recommendations, you should limit your weight loss to 1 to 2 pounds a week. More dramatic reductions are usually due to water and protein loss from the body, while potentially damaging your body as discussed above. Remember that at 1 to 2 pounds a week (eating 500 to 1000 fewer calories a day than you need), you would lose 52 to 104 pounds in a year.

> **NEVER TRY TO LOSE MORE THAN 1-2 POUNDS PER WEEK WITHOUT YOUR DOCTOR'S APPROVAL.**

In the next chapter we are going to look at why "saturated" fat and not dietary cholesterol is responsible for increasing your cholesterol level, leading to heart disease and increasing your risk of stroke.

Chapter Four.
The Truth about Food Labeling and the Food Pyramid.

The labeling of foods is supposed to allow you the consumer to determine what's in a food and how good it is for you. To do this the standard has been to list the serving size (frequently missed or ignored) along with the number of calories per serving. An example of a food label is shown in figure 1.

Figure 1. Example of a food label.

Serving size 1.7 oz. **Calories** 186 Fat Cal. 36		
Amount per serving		% DV
Total Fat:	4 grams	6%
Sat. Fat:	2 grams	10%
Cholesterol:	0 milligrams	0%
Sodium:	63 milligrams	3%
Total carbohydrate:	32 grams	11%
Dietary Fiber:	4 grams	16%
Sugars:	15 grams	
Protein:	5 grams	
% DV is % daily value based on 2000 calorie a day diet.		

Also shown is the total fat, amount of saturated fat, cholesterol, sodium, total carbohydrates – including the dietary fiber and sugars, and the amount of protein per serving. All of the percentages are based upon one serving in relationship to a 2000 calorie (200 pound person x 10 calories/day/pound) a day diet. Of particular interest is the amount of "saturated" and "total" fat present. While this doesn't tell you how much polyunsaturated or monosaturated fat is present, you can figure out how much "polyunsaturated" and "monosaturated" fat you have altogether. In the above example there are 4 grams of total fat of which 2 grams are "saturated" fat. This means that the other 2 grams must be a combination of the "monosaturated" and "polyunsaturated" fats. It also means that 1/2 of the fat present is "saturated."

$$1/2 \text{ saturated fat} = \frac{2 \text{ grams saturated fat}}{4 \text{ grams total fat}}$$

One of the problems people frequently have is the inability to ascertain what a serving size is for a given food. This is a common problem for prepackaged foods such as crackers and chips. The package also suggests a recommended daily value for both cholesterol and sodium, neither of which I knew we had established. Interestingly enough, even though we know you need about 0.35 grams of protein/pound/day, there is no nutritional information on food labels regarding the percentage of your recommended protein intake is present in one serving.

> **LEARNING TO READ A FOOD LABEL CAN BE LIKE READING EGYPTIAN HYROGLYPHICS.**

In our current era of marketing where you are encouraged to eat "low fat," "no fat" foods, consumers are usually unaware of what certain terms mean. Table 1 shows the meanings of many of the currently used terms.

Table 1. Commonly used terms found on food labels and packaging.

Commonly used term	What does it mean
Low calorie	40 calories or less
Reduced calorie	25% fewer calories than original form
Light/Lite	1/3 fewer calories or 50% less fat than original form
Low fat	less than 3 grams of fat
Fat free	less than 1/2 gram of fat
Cholesterol free	less than 2 milligrams of cholesterol
Low sodium	less than 140 milligrams of sodium
Sugar free	less than 1/2 gram of sugar
a good source of RDA*	10 - 19%
high or rich source of RDA*	greater than 20%

* RDA = recommended daily allowance

While these terms can be useful in helping to pick out certain food items, they are only a rough guide and do not tell us the specific amount of anything in the packaged food. A good example are the peanut butter ads which state that one brand of peanut butter has no cholesterol. The implication being that the other brands do or might have cholesterol and therefore aren't as good for you. The truth is, peanut butter doesn't have significant cholesterol in it regardless of which brand you buy (now watch, someone will read the book and change this by adding cholesterol to peanut butter), but they're all loaded with fat – even the "low fat" ones.

> **LOWFAT DOESN'T MEAN NO FAT AND IT ALSO DOESN'T MEAN NO CALORIES.**

For example, regular peanut butter has 74% (140 fat calories out of 190 calories) of its calories in the form of fat. Only 20% of these are saturated because peanut oil is almost 50% monosaturated fat. By comparison reduced fat (another term, meaning less fat than the original form) peanut butter has 53% of its calories in fat (100 fat calories out of 190 calories) of which 21% is saturated fat. This means it has fewer fat calories, but the percentage of saturated fat is the same. The number of calories in the regular and reduced fat versions are also the same (it didn't say reduced calories) and the serving size is only 2 tablespoons. How much peanut butter do you put on your sandwiches?

ALL OILS ARE 100% FAT.

Since most people are at least partially confused about the differences in various types of cooking oils, this is a good place to look at the more readily available ones. By the way, all oils are 100% fat, so don't be fooled by the marketing gimmicks used to sell you one versus another. The differences lie in the percents of saturated, monosaturated and polyunsaturated fat present as shown in table 2. It's also important to realize that the serving sizes of oils are extremely small (usually 1 tablespoon) in comparison to how much most of us use.

Table 2. The amount of cholesterol and the types of fats present in various oils.

Type of Oil	Mg* cholesterol per tablespoon	% Sat. Fat	% Monosat. Fat	% Poly. Fat	% Other Fats
Canola	0	6	62	31	1
Safflower	0	9	12	78	1
Sunflower	0	11	20	69	0
Corn	0	13	25	62	0
Peanut	0	13	49	33	5
Olive	0	14	77	9	0
Soybean	0	15	24	61	0
Margarine	0	18	48	29	5
Vegetable shortening	0	26	43	25	6
Cottonseed	0	27	19	54	0
Lard	12	41	47	12	
Beef fat	14	51	44	4	1
Palm oil	0	51	39	10	0
Butter	33	54	30	4	12
Coconut oil	0	77	6	2	15

* = milligrams, Sat = saturated fat, Monosat = monosaturated fat, and Poly = polyunsaturated fat

Many interesting food trends have occurred over the years, attempting to simplify the process of determining which foods can be exchanged for others. The four food groups were the previously proposed National Standard making the assumption that different foods are equal nutritionally, and that all the consumer needs to do is place everything in a nice neat box. The four food groups have been replaced with the "Food Pyramid." This should not be confused with the original pyramids, even though the proponents of the food pyramid would like you to associate the strength and durability of the pyramids with their food scheme. Interestingly enough, our grandparents and great-grandparents did a much better job of eating the right types and amounts of foods without using such food-exchange programs. While I applaud the efforts of those involved, I would like to point out some of the potential problems you can get into by using such an approach.

THE DIET MYTH

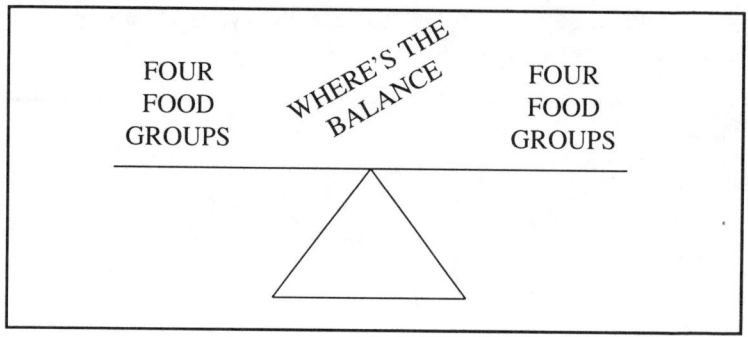

To illustrate these problems lets first look at the food pyramid. At the bottom are the foods listed as breads, cereals, rice and pasta. The guide suggests anywhere from 6 to 11 servings in this group. The second layer is divided into the vegetable group (3 to 5 servings) and the fruit group (2 to 4 servings). Aesthetically this is pleasing because we associate fruits and vegetables as good foods which belong together. In the third tier are the milk, yogurt and cheese group (2 to 3 servings), and the meat, poultry, fish, dry beans, eggs and nuts group (2 to 3 servings) and finally at the peak of the pyramid are the fats, oils and sweets (these are food groups?) group which we are advised to use, sparingly (?).

The problem with this type of arrangement is that it doesn't take into account differences between foods in each of these groups nor is it likely that people are going to devote this pyramid to memory. I don't even want to get into the debates about whether corn is a grain or vegetable. Since we know that the amount of calories, percentages of fat (particularly saturated fat), carbohydrates and protein we need to eat are important in determining our risk of certain health problems, I thought it might be interesting to compare two different dietary regimens using the food pyramid and compare the results with what we know to be important.

The first person in our example is going to eat the following foods for one day: 2 eight ounce glasses of skim milk, 1 skinless chicken breast, 1 ninety-seven percent fat-free hot dog, 1/4 cup of broccoli, 1/4 cup of mixed vegetables, 1/4 cup of black-eyed peas, one medium peach and plum, 2 slices of whole wheat bread, 1 ounce of taboule mix, 2 ounces of elbow macaroni, 1/4 cup of California brown rice and 2 ounces of vermicelli. The second person is going to have 2 eight ounce glasses of whole milk, 1 chicken drumstick, a beef hot-dog, 1/4 cup of corn, 1/4 cup of refried beans, and 1/2 cup of green peas, one-half cup of fruit cocktail and raisins, 1 bagel, a slice of Italian bread, 1 cup of bow tie noodles, 2 ounces of rice pilaf, 2-1/2 ounces of Spanish rice and 2 ounces of lasagna noodles. Doesn't this sound like an interesting way to determine which foods you're going to eat for the day. In our example we're erring on the low side of each number of servings for each group of foods. This should <u>minimize</u> the differences between the two examples.

THE DIET MYTH

Table 3. The food pyramid – the <u>first</u> example (person).

Food Item	How much	Cal.	Fat (gms)	Sat Fat (gms)	Carb (gms)	Prot (gms)	Chol (mg)
Dairy							
skim milk	8 oz	86	0.4	0.3	11.9	8.7	4
skim milk	8 oz	86	0.4	0.3	11.9	8.7	4
Meats							
chicken breast	one	140	1.5	0	0	29	75
97 % fat free hot dog	one	50	1.5	0.5	4	6	20
Veg.							
broccoli	1/4 cup	6	0.05	0	1.3	0	0
mixed veg	1/4 cup	25	0.1	0	5.6	0.4	0
black eyed peas	1/4 cup	50	0.2	0.1	8.6	3.4	0
Fruits							
peach	med	37	0	0	9.2	0	0
plum	med	36	0.4	0.4	8.1	0	0
Grains							
whole wheat	1 slice	70	1.2	0.3	12.5	2.3	0
whole wheat	1 slice	70	1.2	0.3	12.5	2.3	0
taboule mix	1 oz	90	0	0	20	3	0
elbow macaroni	2 oz	210	1	0	40	9	0
Calif. brown rice	1/4 cup	160	1.5	0	34	3	0
vermicelli	2 oz	210	1	0	40	9	0
Totals*		1326	10.45 (94 cal.)	2.2 (21% of total)	219.6 (878 cal)	84.8 (339 cal)	103

* of the 1326 calories, 7% were fat, 67% were carbohydrate and 26% were protein.

Using this same approach we can determine the nutritional value for the food eaten by the second person.

Table 4. The food pyramid – the second attempt.

Food Item	How much	Cal.	Fat (gms)	Sat Fat (gms)	Carb (gms)	Prot (gms)	Chol (mg)
Dairy							
whole milk	8 oz	150	8.2	5.1	11.4	7.6	33
whole milk	8 oz	150	8.2	5.1	11.4	7.6	33
Meats							
chicken drumstick	one	230	12	3	0	27	115
beef hot dog	one	190	17	7	2	6	35
Veg.							
corn	1/4 cup	34	0.05	0	8.4	0	0
refried beans	1/4 cup	104	4	1.6	11	6	6
green peas	1/2 cup	63	0.3	0.1	15	0	0
Fruits							
fruit cocktail	1/2 cup	40	0.1	0	9.8	0	0
raisins	1/4 cup	110	0.2	0.1	28.7	0	0
Grains							
bagel	one	200	1.8	0.3	38.2	7.7	0
Italian bread	1 slice	143	1	0.3	28	5.5	0
bow tie noodles	1 cup	210	1	0	43	7	0
rice pilaf	2 oz	190	0.5	0	42	6	0
Spanish rice	2.5 oz	230	1	0	52	6	0
lasagna noodles	2 oz	210	1	0	40	9	0
Totals		2254 (507 cal)	56.35 40% of total)	22.6 (1363 cal)	340.9 (382 cal)	95.4 mg	222

*of the 2254 calories, 23% were fat, 60% were carbohydrate and 17% are protein.

As you can see, despite adhering to this approach the results were significantly different. In the first example the hypothetical 150 pound person would actually lose 1/3 pound in a week, while the second person would gain 1-1/2 pounds. If the food pyramid approach is designed to be a guide, there could easily be problems with unexpected weight gain following it. Additionally, while the first person did pretty well carbohydrate wise, the amount of protein greatly exceeded their needs, and the amount of fat was too low for the individual's requirements, even though the saturated fat was not a problem. The second person not only gained weight, but ate more than 5-1/2 times the amount of fat (56 grams versus 10 grams) the first person ate, despite the fact that they were both using the same (Food Pyramid) system.

A BALANCED APPROACH SHOULD BE CONSISTENT.

All this using the same method doesn't suggest that this approach will be very useful and if you're looking at cholesterol, the second person ate more than twice what the first person ate. The second person ended up with more protein than the first (they both ate too much), more fat, more saturated fat, and more calories. The percent of carbohydrates eaten were also less. These are the very types of problems we're trying to avoid. If anything the pyramid may represent a rough carbohydrate guide, like most exchange programs, but it didn't work very well for calories, protein, fat or saturated fat.

In the next chapter we're going to discuss the myths of vegetarian diets, their potential benefits and limitations along with other misconceptions present in today's media.

Chapter Five.
The Vegetarian Myth, the Role of *Stress*, Blood Types, Your Horoscope and Hormones for Sale.

Despite the potential health advantages of a more vegetarian lifestyle, people seem to be more divided over the issue of killing something for food rather than the issue of whether it's healthy or not. In the true sense of what is living, even eating a plant could be considered killing something, raising philosophical questions about eating anything. Clearly, a vegetarian existence (whatever that is – table 1) can result in a healthy life as shown by countless individuals who have lived long, healthy lives as vegetarians. The opposite is also true, that not being a vegetarian doesn't mean you will die at an early age. The main truth isn't whether you eat meat, but whether you're eating the right amount of calories, protein, carbohydrates and non-saturated fats.

Table 1. The five major types of vegetarians.

semi-vegetarian	eat dairy, eggs, chicken, fish, no other animal meat
pesco-vegetarian	eat dairy, eggs, fish, no chicken or other animal meat
lacto-ovo-vegetarian	eat dairy foods anad eggs, no other animal meat
ovo-vegetarian	eat eggs, but no dairy or other animal meat
vegan	no animal meat

Becoming a vegetarian doesn't mean you're eating healthy. A primary problem lies in the number of calories many vegetarians are eating. Remember that if you're eating more calories than you need, these extra calories get turned into fat (triglycerides) as shown in figure 1, and this fat can increase your cholesterol and triglyceride levels leading to heart disease, cancer, strokes, obesity and diabetes.

Figure 1. Too many calories regardless of the source become fat.

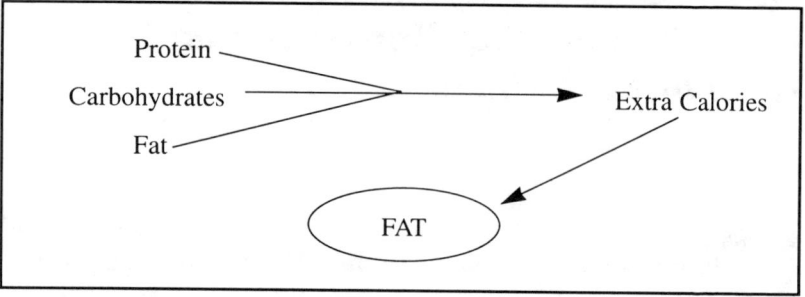

Modern medicine is not the only reason why people are living as long as they do today. If you were a 40-year-old Caucasian male alive in 1910, you would live about as long as a 40-year-old Caucasian male would today. Most of today's healthcare dollars aren't spent on preventing disease, but rather in dealing with the terminal effects of diseases that could have been prevented. In 1997, $1 Trillion (that's right TRILLION) was spent on healthcare (more than 14% of the gross national product) with only 4% of that money going towards the prevention of disease. Yet for every dollar spent on prevention we save $4-10, not to mention the human factor of pain and suffering. It is easy to not spend money on prevention when no one is suffering, but is this the healthiest approach? The current medical model (for many reasons) is focused on a fix-it approach and not a prevent it approach.

> **$1 TRILLION WAS SPENT ON HEALTHCARE IN 1997, ONLY 4% WENT TOWARD THE PREVENTION OF DISEASE.**

The need for a strictly vegetarian life-style has not been shown to be necessary to reverse coronary artery disease or any other health problem. The Tarahumara Indians of Mexico have long been shown to have few health problems including coronary artery (heart) disease. The amount of fat, cholesterol and carbohydrates eaten daily is very similar (table 2) to what Americans and Europeans ate in 1910. The Tarahumara diet consists mainly of corn and beans, fruits and vegetables, and small amounts of wild game, fish and eggs. This means that they are clearly not vegetarians. Their diet consisted of 15% protein, 65% carbohydrates and 20% fat, of which only 1/3 is saturated fat. In the early 1990s a study showed that these same people, when fed an affluent Western diet for 5 weeks, went on to show a 30% increase in their cholesterol levels, a 40% increase in their "bad" cholesterol, and an almost 20% increase in their fat (triglyceride) levels. These people also showed a 7% weight gain in only 5 weeks.

Table 2. Percent of calories consumed as fat, carbohydrate and protein in 1910 and today.

Year	% Fat Calories	% Carbohydrate Calories	% Protein Calories
1910	32	56	12
Today	43	46	11

While we are concerned about increases in cholesterol and triglyceride levels, we are concerned because of the increased potential for heart attacks and strokes. Figures 2, 3 and 4 show the results of three studies looking at maximum blood flow through the different arteries of the heart of a 41-year-old man. Each of the images show the tip of the heart at the center of the image, with the top of the heart at the 12 o'clock position, the bottom part of the heart at 6 o'clock, the outer wall at 3 o'clock and the inner wall at the 9 o'clock position. Blood flow is best where there is red, less when there is yellow and poorest where there is green-black.

This 41-year-old gentleman, husband and father of three, had the first (figure 2 and 3) two studies done 104 days (less than 15 weeks) apart. Like the Tarahumara Indians, who got worse in five weeks on a Western Diet, this gentleman showed a worsening of blood flow

THE DIET MYTH

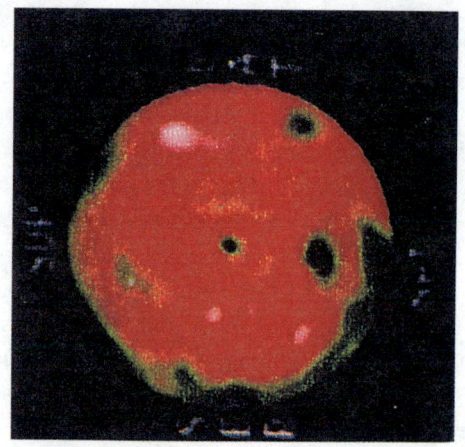

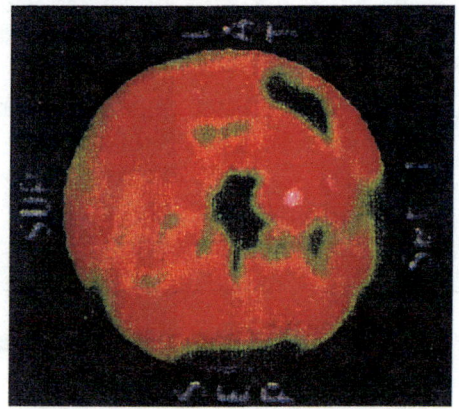

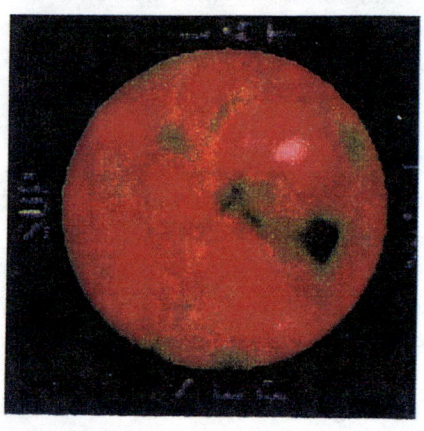

Figure 2, 3 & 4

(increase in disease in the arteries of his heart) in as little as 15 weeks.

His angiogram (dye injected into the arteries of the heart) failed to detect the disease and he continued to eat his usual diet. For this gentleman, less than 4 months time had lead to a significant increase in the disease present in the first artery (7 o'clock position) and the development of new disease in a second artery (4 o'clock) and potentially a third artery at the tip of his heart.

Because of his chest pain and heart disease he was started on medications and placed on the recommended diet (figure 5) to help lower his cholesterol and triglyceride levels. Approximately 4 months later a third study (figure 4) was completed which showed improvement in the blood flow throughout much of his heart.

Figure 5. Recommended diet for healthy living.

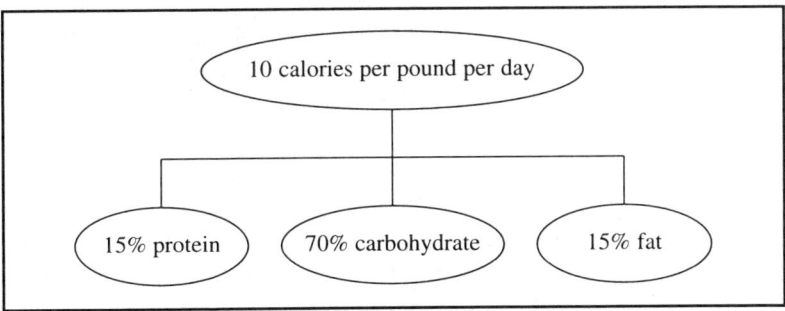

As mentioned earlier in the book, healthy eating is not an issue of sitting in the forest eating tree bark, instead it is an issue of how many calories you're eating daily, and how much of these are fat, saturated fat, carbohydrate and protein.

ALL THIS TALK ABOUT *STRESS* IS *STRESSING ME OUT*

In the 1960s when we began to talk about stress and heart disease it was noticed that there were two different groups of people. This is like looking at food groups, people just love to classify things by groups, and physicians are no exception. The first group we called "Type A" personality and the latter group "Type B." "Type A" represented people who were fairly aggressive (the politically correct term is assertive) and highly driven, competitive individuals. "Type B" people are more relaxed and easy going. The original information suggested that the "Type A" person was more prone to heart disease than the "Type B" person.

> **TYPE A, TYPE B.**
> **TO "B" OR NOT TO "B."**
> **THAT IS THE QUESTION.**

The idea behind this initial information was that "Type A" people were at greater risk because they probably had higher levels of stress hormones in their blood which could cause the heart rate and blood pressure to increase, while increasing the clotting tendency of the blood, and who knew what else. No one is doubting the significance of the effects of these stress hormones, and hopefully no one is suggesting we *all* start taking antidepressant or anti-anxiety medications to deal with our *stressful lives.*

The problem with the initial study was that the people examined were primarily executive men who were constantly under high stress situations, which proved to be harmful to some of them. After more information (and after a book had already been published) it became obvious that "Type A" behavior wasn't significantly worse than "Type B" behavior. The problem occurred when someone was forced to be something they were not. For example, many of the men in the original study were "Type B" people who were forced to live "Type A" lifestyles to survive in their business world. It was this group of people who were at higher risk for heart disease. Similarly, "Type A" people who were forced to become more relaxed (probably to reduce the stress on the "Type B" people around them) were also being forced to be something they are not, and they too appear to be at increased risk. This changed behavior pattern is now called "Type D," which refers to individuals who are exhibiting a different type of behavior than they appear to be "wired" for. Sometimes change is good, sometimes change can be bad!

TYPE "D" BEHAVIOR
BEING WHAT YOU'RE NOT.

Despite all this talk about stress and all the books, radio and television programs designed to show us how we need to change our lifestyle to become more like the "Type B" person, there are no scientific reports showing decreased blood flow to the heart or anywhere else as a result of personality type. There are also no reports showing different eating habits for people of different personality "Types." We're not suggesting that "road rage" is healthy or that any other form of aggressive behavior is good, but "Type A" behavior in and of itself does not appear to cause heart disease and living on a commune in and of itself does not prevent heart disease – or anything else for that matter.

The psychological community has experienced this same phenomena where body types (ectomorph, endomorph and mesomorphic individuals) were thought by some to be indicative of your personality type. There was no scientific proof to support this nonsense either. Nor is there any scientific data to support the idea that your blood type determines the type of food your body needs. You still need a certain number of calories, carbohydrates, protein and fat (linoleic acid). Blood types including A, B, AB and O (these are the major blood types, there are other factors) have nothing more to do with the type of food you should be eating than does your horoscope. Regardless of what you think of horoscopes, they are not nutritional guides. In fact, the blood type issue and horoscopes have a lot in common. They are both so vague that they include everybody and nobody at the same time. The more vague you get (blood types, horoscopes, et cetera), the more credit you can take for getting something right and the more you can deny something you were wrong about. Most people would like someone else to assume (at least part of the) responsibility for their problems (health or anything else). I think figure 6 just about sums up this approach.

Finally, one of the newest trends to hit the "diet" and "health" market are THE HORMONES. You would think that with all the known side effects of birth control pills (increased blood clots, decreased levels of vitamins B-6, B-12, folate, riboflavin, C and zinc, along with increases in vitamin A [blindness] and copper) that it would be more difficult to con so many people. But WHERE THERE'S A DOLLAR, THERE'S A WAY, particularly when the Food and Drug Administration (FDA) doesn't have the ability to control these substances (non-prescription hormones, vitamins and minerals) like they do prescription medications written by "Medical Doctors." From the government's perspective this is like buying toothpaste.

The four most popular include Dehydroepiandrosterone (DHEA) which is sold as something which will increase your sex drive (a common theme for these hormones and probably what most people buy them for), and improve your immune function and muscle strength. What it may actually do is increase your risk of breast and ovarian cancer if you're a woman, or prostate cancer if you're a man. Alternatively, there's Testosterone (male hormone), again promoted to increase your sex drive (do you think these people are obsessed with this) and muscle tone, but may also increase your risk of heart disease. Then there's Pregnenolone advertised to improve your memory and reduce fatigue (wouldn't we all like that) but has no real proof to back it up, but since the body changes it to DHEA, it comes with the risk for cancer. Finally there is Melatonin, marketed as the miracle cure to stop aging and the jet lag cure – works for some not all. The study which suggested the anti-aging effect was discredited, although it may cause strokes by narrowing arteries to the brain and decrease your fertility. So I guess the DHEA could be taken to help with possible side effects from the Melatonin.

Figure 6. If only I could blame something other than what I'm eating. The role of denial.

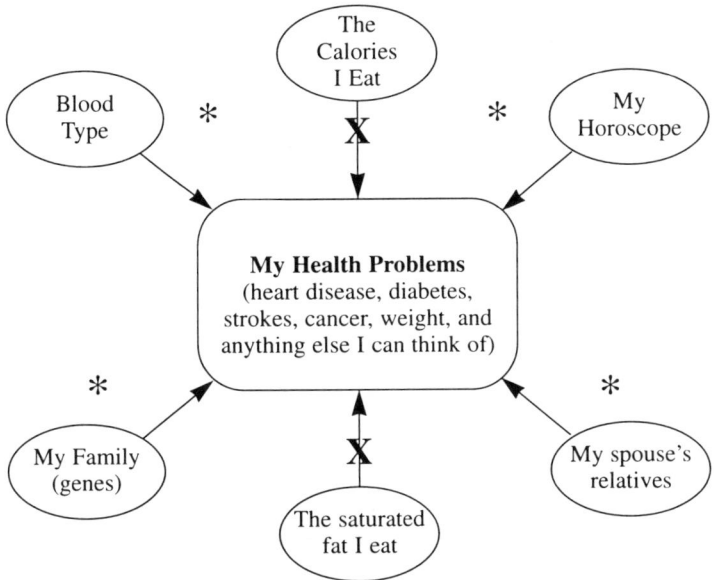

X = this could be my fault, this couldn't be the problem
* - this is a great idea, I can't be held accountable for this

Chapter Six.
What's all the Confusion about Cholesterol?

You have undoubtedly heard more about cholesterol during the last 20 to 30 years than you ever wanted to. Because of the mass confusion all this has produced, I thought it might be helpful to talk about how the medical system works, and then to clear up the confusion. Once a year the American College of Cardiology (ACC) holds a national meeting in the Spring, and once a year the American Heart Association (AHA) does the same in the Fall. During these meetings (as well as others held throughout the world) research is presented for discussion and review. Most of this is preliminary work that will <u>never</u> become part of a medical journal. Most of it will soon be forgotten, except by the media, who will try their best to cover what they assume is the latest-breaking information.

The purpose of these meetings isn't to confuse anybody, but to increase our interest in research and discuss heart disease. (By the way, the other medical sciences are doing the same thing.) If, after the preliminary work has been done, there is any reason to continue further investigation, some additional work may be done and presented at still another meeting. Over time something may get published after the medical editors (like myself) of a journal have reviewed and corrected it. If the information stands the test of time, it may become part of a textbook to teach young (and hopefully older) doctors what they need to know to treat their patients. As you can see, there is a big difference between talking about something and considering it worth being part of medical practice.

> **SOMETIMES WE GET MORE MISINFORMATION THAN USEFUL INFORMATION.**

Because cholesterol and heart disease are so important, many people are interested in learning more about it and so the race for information (and sometimes misinformation) continues. (This is where I would normally draw a picture of several doctors running around a track, chasing something called cholesterol. Unfortunately my talents don't include drawing people – but you get the picture.)

WHERE DOES THE CHOLESTEROL IN MY BODY COME FROM?

Cholesterol primarily comes from one of two sources: the <u>first</u> is the food you eat, and the <u>second</u> is what your liver makes. Animals and plants are different in many ways, including the production of cholesterol. Since animals make cholesterol it should not be surprising that the foods we eat with the greatest amount of cholesterol include meats, dairy and animal products. The parts of our bodies that have the most cholesterol are the parts of the animals' bodies which have the most cholesterol: heart, liver, brains, kidneys, meat – dark meat more than white meat – and the skin. As you may have already guessed, most of the cholesterol found in animals (including people) is not found in their blood, but throughout the rest of their body. Likewise, only 7% of our cholesterol is found in our blood, while the other 93% is stored elsewhere.

> **93% OF YOUR CHOLESTEROL ISN'T IN YOUR BLOOD.**

Some animals have more cholesterol than others (table 1), and as we've already discussed, trimming away the fat reduces the saturated fat but not the cholesterol. As seen in figure 1, there is no relationship between the amount of cholesterol and the amount of fat present in something. For example, shrimp which has almost no fat is relatively high in cholesterol. Most of the different types of meat we eat have between 60 and 90 milligrams of cholesterol per 3 ounce serving, while the amount of fat ranges between 1/2 and 11 grams.

Table 1. Cholesterol and fat grams for 3 ounce servings of different meats.

Animal	Milligrams of Cholesterol	Grams of Fat
Shrimp	166	0.9
Veal	128	4.7
Oysters	93	4.2
Blue crab	85	1.5
Pork	79	11.1
Dark (skinless) chicken	79	8.2
Lamb	78	8.8
Beef	77	8.7
Salmon	74	9.3
Dark (skinless) turkey	72	6.1
White (skinless) chicken	72	3.8
Lobster	61	0.5
White (skinless) turkey	59	1.3
Scallops	34	0.8

The average Western diet includes 250 to 500 milligrams of cholesterol daily. Of this, only about 10% will actually enter your body. This means that of what you're eating, only about 25 to 50 milligrams are absorbed daily. Your liver is busily making 1000 milligrams each and every day. If you eat more cholesterol, your liver simply adjusts to this, making less if you eat more and making more if you eat less. This is because your liver is responsible for making sure your body has all the cholesterol it needs to make cell membranes and hormones.

Figure 1. There is no relationship between the amount of cholesterol and fat in a meat.

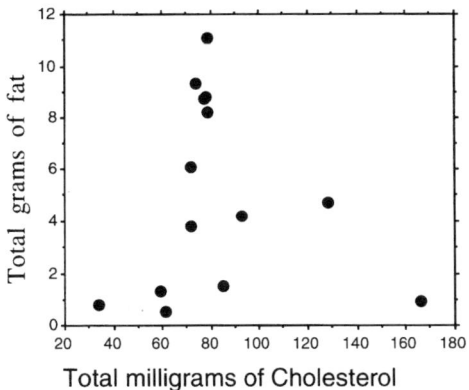

Studies looking at the amount of cholesterol in your diet and your blood cholesterol level have been contradictory and you have been hearing one story one year and something else the next. Whenever this happens you should be suspicious that the whole story isn't known or isn't being reported. Blood cholesterol is more dependent upon the excess calories and saturated fat eaten than the amount of cholesterol in the diet (see table 2).

Table 2. What foods change cholesterol levels.

Food	Effect upon cholesterol
Excess calories	increases
Saturated fat	increases
Monosaturated fat	no effect*
Polyunsaturated fat	decreases*

* assuming one is not eating too many calories

THE PROOF'S IN THE PUDDING (SO TO SPEAK)

In the early 1990s we began looking at the differences between dietary change and medications and how these effected cholesterol and triglyceride (fat) levels. Since we had already helped establish the reversibility of heart disease, we were now trying to determine what we were doing right and what we were doing wrong. Despite the belief by many people, that you have to become vegetarian to reverse heart disease, we discovered something completely different, or <u>at least we thought it was different</u>.

The first group of people we studied followed the Nationally Recommended guidelines of lowering the amount of cholesterol eaten in a day to 250 mg or less. These people showed an average increase in cholesterol of 18% over 18 months. People who reduced the number of calories they ate to 10 calories/pound/day and who reduced the amount of saturated fat eaten, showed a 40% reduction in cholesterol during the first six months, or 60% if they were also taking cholesterol lowering medicines. The improvement continued as long as they followed these dietary habits.

> **CHANGING THE DIET REDUCED CHOLESTEROL LEVELS 40 - 60%.**

Figure 2 shows how blood flow to the heart improved in one person, 1 year after following the dietary guidelines outlined in figure 3. This blood flow study like those shown elsewhere in the book, show the tip of the heart at the center of each image. The top part of the heart is at 12 o'clock, the bottom part at 6 o'clock, the outer wall at 3 o'clock and the inner wall at 9 o'clock. The best blood flow is represented by red, with orange, yellow, green, and blue representing less and less blood flow, while black represents no blood flow. The top two pictures show the resting (left) and maximal (right) blood flow to the heart when the person entered the study. The bottom two images show the results one year later with resting blood flow on the left and maximum blood flow on the right. Twelve months after changing her diet, her blood flow was better to the top and bottom of her heart.

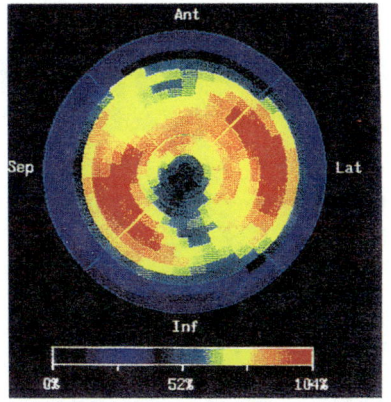
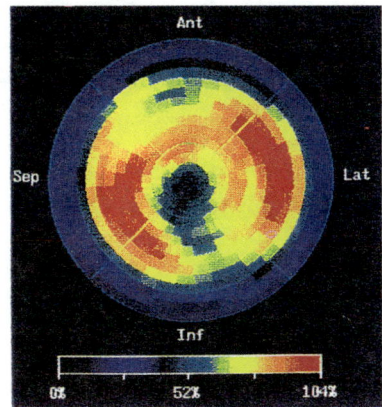
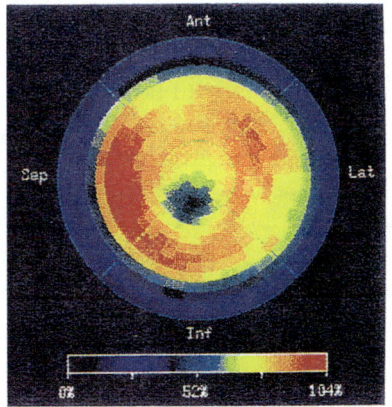
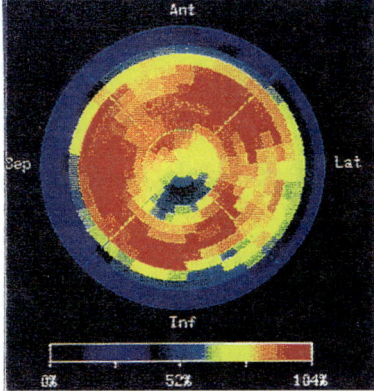

Figures 2

Figure 3. Recommended diet for healthy living.

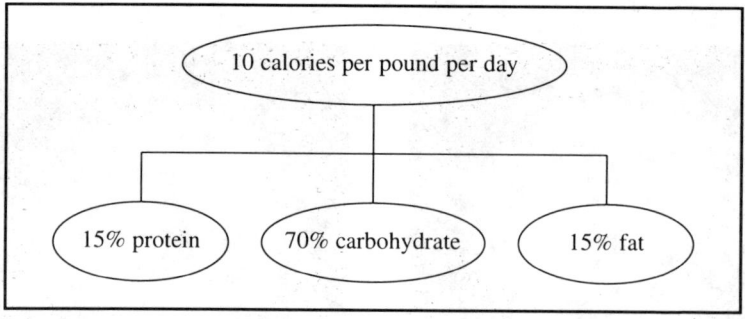

What our research has shown is that the key to reducing cholesterol levels, is not linked to the amount of cholesterol you eat, but the amount of saturated fat, and excess calories you're eating. The problem is that many foods with relatively high cholesterol levels tend to be those with relatively high saturated fat. These excess calories and saturated fats get turned into body fat (triglycerides) and in the liver (figure 4) helps drive cholesterol production. While I wish I could say I was the first to discover this, I cannot. A gentleman by the name of Ancel Keys was the first to point out the relationship between saturated fat and elevated cholesterol levels. We were just fortunate enough to show improvement in blood flow to the heart with the avoidance of "bad" foods, while eating the right types of food.

Figure 4. The production of cholesterol from excess calories and saturated fat.

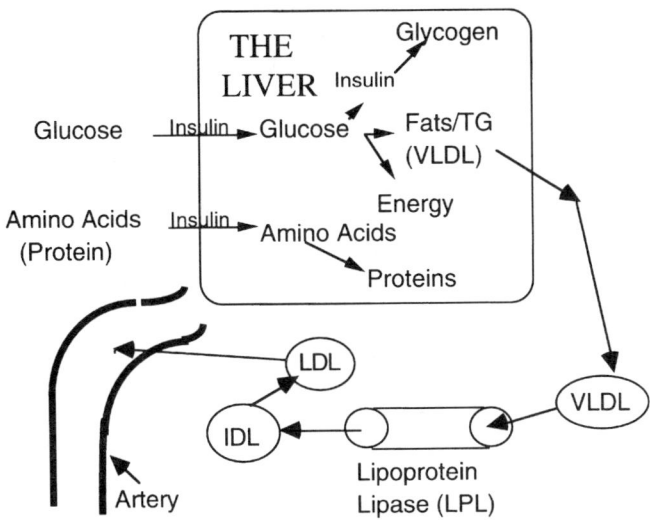

As we have already seen, extra calories (figure 4) get turned into fat (triglycerides). The liver uses this to make very-low density lipoprotein cholesterol (VLDL) which is changed in the blood vessels of our body into intermediate density lipoprotein cholesterol (IDL) by an enzyme called lipoprotein lipase (LPL). The IDL is rapidly changed to low-density lipoprotein (LDL) cholesterol, which we have come to know as "bad cholesterol." It is this LDL cholesterol which builds up in the arteries of our heart leading to heart attacks. In addition to too many calories and saturated fat in our diets, there are several medical problems which can cause higher than desirable levels of triglycerides (fat). Many of these are shown in table 3 and should be discussed with your doctor when considering treatment.

Table 3. Other factors which increase triglyceride (VLDL) levels which can lead to increases in cholesterol levels.

Alcohol
Beta-blocking medications
Diabetes Mellitus
Diuretic medications
Estrogens (female hormones)
Excessive calories
Glucocorticoid medications
Hypothyroidism (too little thyroid)
Nephrotic syndrome (kidney problem)
Obesity
Pancreatitis
Pregnancy
Primary Biliary Cirrhosis

Along with dietary change and medications which can reduce the liver's ability to make LDL cholesterol, there is a new medication available in the United States this year (1998) which can lower your body's ability to make triglycerides. This medicine has been successfully used for years in Europe and Canada and is called **fenofibrate.**

> **CHOLESTEROL AND TRIGLYCERIDE LEVELS OVER 150 SHOULD BE CONSIDERED HIGH.**

In the end we are what we eat. If we eat more calories than we need, or too much saturated fat, we're going to make additional cholesterol to deposit in our bodies. All of this results in more heart disease, strokes, diabetes, obesity and some forms of cancer. Regardless of who we are and what we're concerned with, changes in our diets have lead to more health problems in the United States, Europe, developing countries, and yes even people like the Tarahumara Indians of Mexico. In the next chapter we are going to look at how several issues are adding to the risk of stroke and heart disease, and what we may be able to do to prevent them.

Chapter Seven.
What's Causing Heart Disease and Strokes?

If you're thinking that everything you've heard about cholesterol and heart disease cannot possibly explain why Uncle Fred doesn't have heart disease despite eating everything bad known to man, smoking like a chimney and setting the *Guinness Book of Records* for most hours sitting in an easy chair – YOU'RE RIGHT!!! Heart disease isn't just due to one thing and the amount of cholesterol you eat – as you have been reading – isn't the key either.

Doctors are trained to look for the "risk factors" of heart disease when someone develops chest pain and it sounds like it's coming from the heart. The typical risk factors (table 1) help to guestimate whether someone might have heart disease. I'm always astounded when someone has just had a heart attack and the doctor say's he/she shouldn't have had one because they don't have any risk factors; their cholesterol doesn't seem high enough, they don't smoke (anymore), they exercise regularly, and they don't have a family history of heart disease. Risk factors suggest the "risk" that a problem might occur, but once you've had the problem, the chance (probability) is 100% – that's as high as it gets!

When I was with the Iowa Heart Association, we were developing a program called "Don't Stall Call 911" designed to encourage people to call an ambulance for help getting them (or their loved one) to the hospital where they could get treatment if they needed it. The interviews of couples were interesting to watch. People who had already had either a heart attack, angioplasty (balloon procedure to widen a narrowed artery) or bypass operation (veins placed above and below narrowed artery to improve blood flow) were asked if the pain they were having was the same as the pain they had before when they were having heart problems. Almost everyone would say YES. When asked if they thought the new pain (identical to their prior heart pain) could be from their heart they would almost always say NO. Their spouse (husband or wife) would always look at them to say "you're kidding." What we learned from this was the level of denial someone could have when they were worried that their pain was coming from their heart. It is the spouse/loved one/significant other who gets the person to the hospital.

Table 1. Conventional risk factors for heart disease.

Prior heart problems	If you've had it before and it's the same, you're having it again.
Lack of estrogen	You're either a male or a women without ovarian function.
Smoking	Increases heart rate, blood pressure and makes your blood want to clot.
Hypertension (High blood pressure)	The higher your blood pressure the the harder your heart has to work.
Diabetes Mellitus	If you're diabetic your blood vessels and nerves don't work as well as they should.
Obesity	The more you weigh the more work your heart has to do.
High levels of "bad" cholesterol.	Whether due to too many saturated fats or too many calories, this stuff likes to deposit itself in the arteries of your body.
High triglyceride (fat) levels	Where the fats (VLDL) are high, the ability to make more bad (LDL) cholesterol appears to increase.

I remember when I was a resident physician, I had a woman in the emergency room with left ear pain. Someone else had gotten an electrocardiogram (ECG) to look at her heart. The ECG was essentially normal and this woman's left ear was red just like it should be if she had an ear infection. For some reason, I can't explain why, I admitted her to the Coronary Care Unit (CCU) for observation. I felt pretty stupid at the time, but the results of her blood work showed us she had already had a "small" heart attack and her only clue was her left ear pain. As I tell my residents, if the pain someone has is identical to that which they had before when they were having heart problems, admit them to the hospital and assume it's their heart – no matter how strange the pain sounds.

Another risk factor for heart disease is the lack of estrogen. This female hormone may provide some benefit although younger and younger women are having problems with heart disease and heart attacks. When women stop having menstrual cycles (menopause, surgery, birth control) they have an increased risk of heart disease. The safest approach appears to be estrogen patches or possibly soybeans which have a plant-like hormone similar to estrogen.

> **WOMEN ARE HAVING HEART DISEASE AT YOUNGER AND YOUNGER AGES.**

Smoking is clearly another risk for heart disease and strokes. The problem with smoking is it's difficult to stop for many people once they've started. Ignoring many of the problems other people are talking about, smoking releases chemicals into your blood stream which cause your heart rate and blood pressure to increase, thereby causing your heart to work harder. It also makes the blood want to stick together more, leading to the potential for blood clots. There's nothing you need less than a blood clot floating through an already narrowed artery.

> **SMOKING INCREASES YOUR HEART RATE, BLOOD PRESSURE AND MAKES YOUR BLOOD WANT TO CLOT.**

Hypertension (high blood pressure) makes your heart work harder. This is like taking all the water lines to a city and making them smaller while expecting the water pump downtown (or where ever it is) to pump the same amount of water everywhere it had before. To do this, you need a bigger pump. For the heart to do this, it must get thicker, and this, in and of itself, increases the potential for a heart attack. The smaller water lines for the city and its pump are similar to arteries clogged with cholesterol. Usually, the arteries don't all narrow or clog up at the same rate, and the blood from the heart goes where there is the least resistance. This means the diseased (narrowed or plugged up) arteries receive less blood flow. Whatever these arteries supply becomes deprived of oxygen and food; for example, if the arteries of your neck narrow, you might have a stroke, if the artery goes to one of your legs you might lose a leg, or have a heart attack if the artery goes to your heart.

> **HIGH BLOOD PRESSURE MAKES YOUR HEART WORK HARDER.**

If you have diabetes mellitus (there's also a diabetes insipidus – totally different problem) the smaller blood vessels of your body are affected resulting in problems with your nerves functioning correctly. For example, if you're a diabetic individual and you stand up too quickly your heart rate may not be able to correct for the drop in your blood pressure. As a result you may faint. Over time the arteries which bother diabetic people the most are those in their eyes, because it can cause blindness (diabetic retinopathy). People with diabetes also have problems with high cholesterol and triglyceride (fat) levels which by themselves increase their risk of heart disease.

Obesity raises some of the same concerns as high blood pressure. Since you only have one pump (your heart) if you increase the amount of your body which needs to receive food and oxygen from it, you have increased the work load on your heart. If a city had a water pump which adequately supplied water to ten thousand homes, and another ten thousand homes were added, the original water pump wouldn't be able to keep up with the demand and either everyone would end up without water or they would have less water than they needed to eat, drink, bath, wash clothes, et cetera.

If you lived in one of the original ten thousand homes (or even one of the newer ones) and the city did this to you without adding a new pump, you would probably get very upset with the city government. Yet people don't get upset with themselves or cut back on the calories and saturated fat they are eating to reduce their weight which overburdens their hearts. Instead we tend to buy into diet gimmicks and fads which don't solve the problem, but makes us feel like we're doing something about it, even though we're not.

> **IF THE GOVERNMENT DID TO YOU WHAT YOU DO TO YOU, YOU'D BE UPSET. SO WHY AREN'T YOU?**

High levels of "bad" cholesterol (LDL greater than 100 mg/dl) and high triglyceride (fat) levels (greater than 200 and probably anything greater than 150 mg/dl) result in a build-up in the arteries of our body on a gradual day-by-day basis. All of the arteries in our body can be affected even though most of the attention has been on the heart. Clearly the brain, gut, kidneys, legs and other parts of the body can also be damaged.

These eight factors aren't the only risk factors for heart disease although they're usually the ones we talk about. People whose parents, grandparents, aunts and uncles, have had heart disease may be at a greater risk for heart disease. The risk is thought to increase if, and only if, family members had problems (heart pain/heart attacks) when they were younger than 55 years of age. The reason for this is clear from our research. Most of us will increase our cholesterol levels an average of 2% each and every year assuming we make no changes in what we are currently eating or the medications we are taking. Given this information, most of us will have elevated cholesterol and triglyceride levels by age 55, if not before. So a family history doesn't mean you have to be at increased risk, simply that you might be. The reason for this may be as simple as the way you were taught to eat or the lifestyle you live versus any genetic tendency.

> **THE WAY YOU LEARN TO EAT MAY BE THE MOST IMPORTANT RISK FACTOR YOUR FAMILY GIVES YOU.**

While the above factors may suggest an increased potential for heart disease and strokes, they do not in and of themselves mean that you will have problems, and just like I ask my medical students, if you have none of these risk factors but you just had a heart attack, does that mean you have nothing to worry about?

<u>ARTERIES ARE ARTERIES</u>
&
<u>VEINS ARE VEINS</u>

Arteries are arteries, the only difference is where they go in the body. By the way, arteries and veins are not the same thing. Veins return blood to the heart and are relatively thin walled, while arteries take blood away from the heart and are thicker. If you don't think this is important, and you may not, think about it this way. If you want to go from the United States to Mexico you head south; if you go the other direction you'll end up (eventually) in Canada. The direction you're going from something is important and if you can't get the name of the road right how do you expect to get where you're going. (End of anatomy lesson.)

When people are born, their arteries expand and relax with every beat of the heart. Over time this stretching and relaxing causes minor injuries to the arteries. When "bad" cholesterol levels increase, as a result of excess calories and/or "saturated" fat, this "bad" cholesterol finds these areas of damage. This "bad" cholesterol enters the arteries of your body where it shouldn't be. This only happens if there is too much of the "bad" cholesterol. Your body has other defenses to help you deal with this "bad" cholesterol, including "homocysteine" and antioxidants, both of which try to help repair the damaged artery. However, if your "homocysteine" and/or antioxidants are too low or if your "bad" cholesterol is too high, your arteries cannot be repaired fast enough to prevent the build-up of cholesterol inside them.

Once inside an artery, your body's defense mechanisms (white blood cells) try to remove the cholesterol by eating (phagocytosis) it. This removes the cholesterol from the wall of the artery, but now it's inside the white blood cell, which is itself within the wall of the artery (figure 1).

Chelating agents which are supposed to work by removing calcium (or anything else) do not have time to go through both the wall of the artery and the white blood cell to remove the calcium and cholesterol build-up. There are no scientifically reported studies of chelation reversing heart disease. A different technique called plasmapheresis, removes blood and filters (removes) excess "bad" (LDL) cholesterol from the blood itself, thereby reducing what is available to enter the wall of the artery. Chelation, which means "claw like" attacks or binds itself to a metal, like calcium. It will remove calcium from anyplace it can find it. Since your bones have lots of blood vessels within them, these chelating agents flow right through these rich sources of calcium, removing the calcium from your bones and potentially doing the same thing to the muscles and nerves of your body.

Figure 1. Why chelation doesn't work.

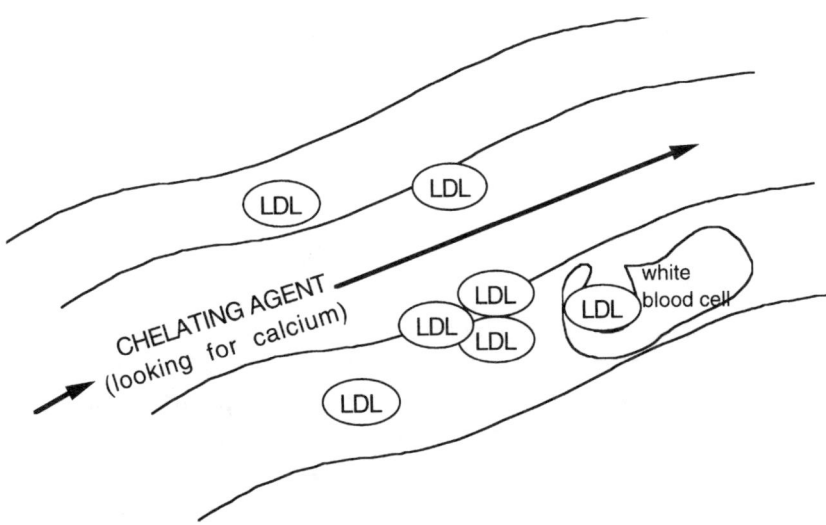

Once these white blood cells (called macrophages) have eaten the "bad/LDL" cholesterol they die and become "foam cells." The build-up of these foam cells over time cause bulges in the arteries which narrow the center part (lumen) of the artery where the blood normally flows. These bulges can break or rupture spilling into the lumen of the artery and, like a cut in you skin, the body will try to close the cut to reduce blood loss. This causes a blood clot to form (figure 2), which may completely block blood flow, leading to a heart attack or stroke. Even if the bulge doesn't rupture, the narrowing itself can cause a blood clot to form.

Figure 2. Blood clot stops blood flow to heart, brain or elsewhere.

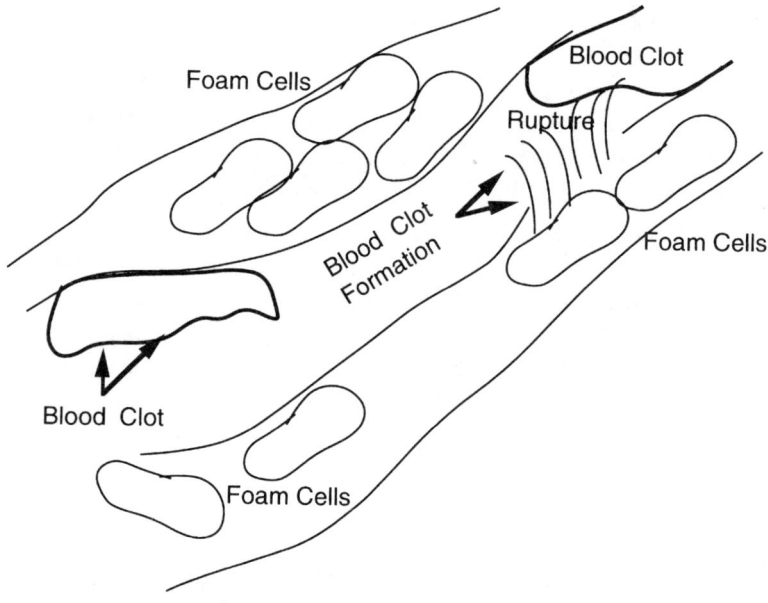

This ability to cause a blood clot in some individuals has been shown to be a problem once the artery has started to narrow. People with too much (clotting factors) fibrinogen or lipoprotein (a) may clot earlier than they should. This is another reason why clotting and blockage of an artery can occur when relatively little narrowing of the artery has occurred. It has been shown that men who have had a heart attack may benefit from taking aspirin daily. This reduces the clotting tendency of the blood, enhancing blood flow in these narrowed, diseased arteries. We do not know (and probably never will) if 81 mg of aspirin, 325 mg of aspirin (normal adult strength) or some other amount/dose is more appropriate since such a study would place someone at risk for a heart attack or stroke.

When something inside your body is damaged, your body's defenses come to your aid. In the case of cholesterol build-up in your arteries, white blood cells called macrophages try to help. In the case of damage and further injury to your arteries, other white blood cells come in to repair the damage along with the macrophages. These other white blood cells (monocytes and PMN's) try to narrow the artery to reduce further blood loss. However, this narrowing can reduce the amount of blood getting through and cause further blood clots. Once the wall of the artery has been damaged, bacteria in the area can enter the artery and cause still more damage. These bacteria have been seen in arteries of both the neck and heart and are somewhat protected from our bodies defenses that would normally kill them.

Figure 3. Fleming Unified Theory of Vascular Disease.

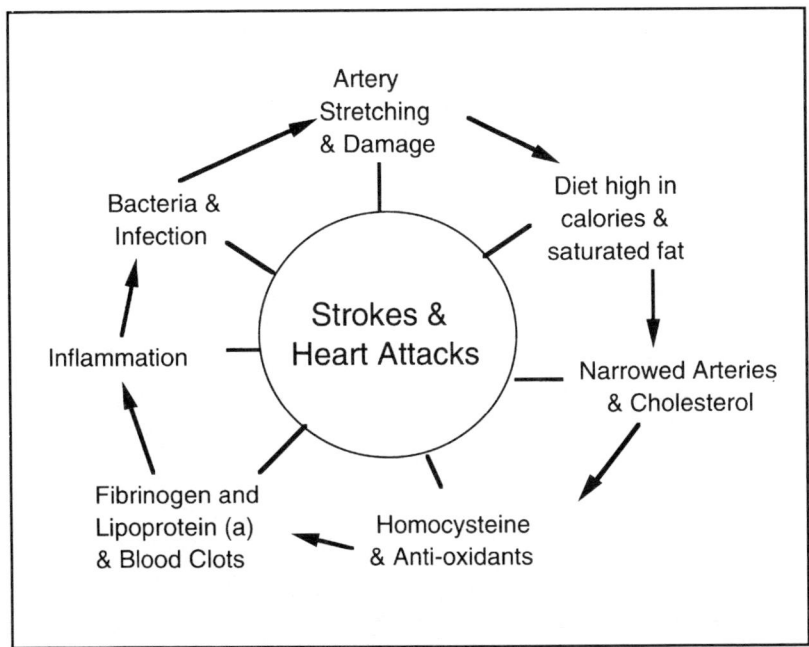

Since we know that one thing can lead to another and our body is trying to compensate for the damage we are doing to it with the foods we are eating, it should be obvious that we can do something about it. Nowhere in the scheme of things do we see any benefit behind extremistic diets or fads. Pills which increase your metabolism along with your heart rate and blood pressure aren't the answer either. Taking megadoses of vitamins to try to slow down the problem won't prevent the inevitable if we continue to abuse our bodies.

Becoming a marathon runner won't help us if we continue to eat garbage. Spending thousands of dollars a year to belong to a health club or spa, won't make us eat better. Becoming a vegetarian (whatever variety) won't keep you from overeating (saturated fats and calories), neither will eliminating carbohydrates and fats which your body needs to be its healthiest. You also don't have to live at the doctors office out of fear.

> **THERE ARE NO GIMMICKS OR FADS WHICH WILL WORK LONGTERM.**

In the end, success is determined by what we decide to do with each situation. There's an old Chinese proverb:

> *"If we don't change the direction we are going,*
>
> *we will end up where we're headed."*

In the next chapter we're going to look at some of the common sense approaches to getting where we want to go, instead of where we're headed.

Chapter Eight.
Common Sense About Losing Weight.

Most men and women today grew up during a time when we ate less and were more active. As a result, we weighed less and felt better. As people get older, they spend less time on their personal appearance and focus more on their careers (either in or outside of the home). As work schedules and family demands increase, most of us spend less time worrying about our bodies until one day we suddenly notice we look and feel different than we did when we were younger.

Faced with the reality of aging bodies we do what most people do – we panic and start to reach for anything that says it will make us healthier, happier, stronger, and stop us from aging. Most people are looking for the Fountain of Youth, or at least the Fountain of Middle-age. Today you can find almost any cosmetic product imaginable and, assuming you have enough time in the day, you could probably use all of them. Many businesses have become profitable by selling products designed to appeal to our egos and sense of self-esteem.

> **MANY BUSINESSES PROFIT BY OUR SEARCH FOR THE FOUNTAIN OF YOUTH.**

Weight loss is no exception to this. Most of the products advertised tell you you will lose "X" amount of weight in "X" amount of time. Time to fit into a new swimsuit, try our product. Unsightly bulges, try our product. Eat more and lose weight, eat more of this, that and the other thing and lose weight. Does it really make sense to anyone that eating more of something will help you lose weight? Isn't this like telling the consumer, that if you shop during a sale you will save a certain amount of money, when in reality you're spending more money than if you didn't go to the sale at all. The idea is to "sell" you on an idea that makes someone else money, and once you're sold, you belong to the person doing the selling and they know it.

The term "cellulite" is a good example of something used to sell books, diet products, and anything else you can be sold. The term "cellulite" has a meaning we've all come to accept, yet it's not present in any of my medical dictionaries or any other dictionary I've looked into. How can you sell a product for something that doesn't exist? I'll tell you how. You write a book or use the term enough to make people think it's real. Place a picture of someone on the cover of the book enough times and say this is what cellulite is and people will accept it. Despite what people try to con you into believing, there are no quick and safe ways to lose weight and keep it off. If there were, someone would have become rich patenting the idea.

CELLULITE: A WORD LOOKING FOR A MEANING.

Fat is deposited in different parts of your body depending upon whether your a man or a woman. Men tend to put it around their waist (abdomen) and women put it around their hips, thighs and upper arms. Women also tend to deposit it throughout their skin, which provides an extra layer for insulation to keep them warmer. The number of fat cells (adipose tissue) you have is primarily determined during your first few years of life. This is why parents who overfeed their children can predispose them to obesity in later years.

You may be asking: if the number of fat cells in your body was at least partially determined by what your parents feed you (it's your parents fault again – right) or didn't feed you (wait a minute, maybe these people actually helped you) during your first few years of life, what can you do about your weight today? Good question! The number of fat cells may be determined at an early age, but you determine how much fat you're going to store there. That's right. The more you eat, the more fat there will be to store in these cells. You might think this sets a limit, but some people work at filling this limit with a vengeance.

> **YOUR FAT CELLS ARE LIKE WAREHOUSES, JUST BECAUSE THEY'RE THERE DOESN'T MEAN YOU HAVE TO FILL THEM ALL THE WAY TO THE TOP.**

The key to losing weight <u>and keeping it off</u> isn't deciding to do something today so you can stop doing it tomorrow. I had a radio talk show host ask me once what I thought of a certain diet he/she was on. I tried to find a way to come up with a positive response since I could see this person was really trying to lose weight. When I finished he/she (notice I don't want to give the gender of the host away) said they couldn't wait to be off the diet because they hated being on it. With this type of an approach, how can anyone possibly be successful at keeping the weight off, assuming they can even lose the weight to begin with.

A number of companies try to find celebrities who will endorse their product because we all want to be like the rich and famous. It makes us feel good about ourselves to say we are doing the same thing as someone else who has been successful, particularly if they've been successful at losing weight. In the end, most of these people find themselves with the same weight and health problems they had before. Another technique used are the pictures of people before and after they follow a diet plan. The before pictures always include clothes meant to make the person look as big as possible. Imagine letting someone talk you into having such a picture taken. Of course you wouldn't know they were trying to make you look overweight. The after picture always tends to be taken on an angle, and with the person wearing clothes that make them look thinner. (Clothes really do make the man, or woman!)

> **THE QUICKEST WAY TO LOOK THINNER IS TO WEAR CLOTHES THAT MAKE YOU LOOK THINNER.**

I live in a city of approximately 750,000 people, but the smallest version of our telephone book had 21 physicians who do Liposuction or "skin sculpting" procedures. The art of looking beautiful on the outside is a big business, but it reminds me of the "body builder" who lifts weights all day to make their muscles big and then dies from a heart attack, because the inside is not in the shape it needs to be.

> **TAKING CARE OF THE OUTSIDE OF YOU DOESN'T HELP THE INSIDE.**

Our bodies are a lot like our personal relationships – if we don't work on them, they deteriorate. Fortunately for our bodies (and our relationships) we can do something about it before it's too late. Some of the greatest advocates for healthy eating come from people who have had a heart attack or have come very close it. Since 1/3 to 1/2 of all heart attacks occur in people with no prior warning signs, waiting until you have a heart attack, seems to me to be the risky approach.

If you're going to try to lose weight, there are certain things you must remember. <u>First</u>, when you put on weight you put in on where your fat cells are. That's why you look the way you do. <u>Second</u>, when you try to lose weight you should try to lose one to two pounds a week. You put it on slowly, you have to take it off slowly to avoid hurting your body. <u>Third</u>, many people who lose weight on these "DIETS" are losing water. You want to make sure this doesn't happen to you. To avoid this water loss and dehydration, drink plenty of water. If you're like most people you think you drink plenty of water but you don't. Try to drink at least 6-8 ten-to-twelve ounce glasses of water each day. If your urine is dark yellow, you're definitely not drinking enough.

> **YOU NEED 6-8 TEN-TO-TWELVE OUNCE GLASSES OF WATER A DAY.**

Fourth, BALANCE NOT EXTREMISM is THE KEY. Forget about the gimmicks and avoid all these diets which have no research to back them up, or you only hear about the first group of people and no one tells you want happens to most of the people who continue on these plans over time. What we're reporting in this book is what has been shown to work in several studies we have done, year after year after year. It worked for our ancestors and it works for people in other parts of the world. More importantly, I'm not calling it the FLEMING DIET, and I don't want you to either. There is no such thing as a FLEMING FOOD GROUP and I don't want one. I'm not selling you a bunch of vitamins and I refuse to sell vitamins and books in my office. I have concerns about people who do and think that the practice of medicine is something similar to a traveling side show from the wild, wild west.

> **YOU SHOULD TRY TO LOSE ONLY 1-2 POUNDS A WEEK TO AVOID HURTING YOUR BODY.**

Fifth, following a balanced approach and eating 500 to 1000 fewer calories than you need each day will result in your loosing 1 to 2 pounds per week. This means that you will be using up fat calories and not ripping apart your muscle and other sources of protein to deal with diet plans which attempt faster weight loss. Most people who lose weight rapidly do so by losing too much water and body protein, in addition to the fat. When you only lose the fat, the protein and water remain where they belong. You also get the additional benefit of not damaging your liver, kidneys, bones, brain, and you don't develop kidney stones or cause your body to be acidotic.

By the way, don't fall for those gimmicks where people have you check your urine to find out how acidic (or alkaline/base) your urine is. This doesn't tell you if you're eating the right foods. Urine

THE DIET MYTH

tends to be acidic unless your kidneys have failed or are damaged. If you let urine sit at room temperature long enough, the bacteria present will change it from an acid to a base. So if you don't like it being acidic (this is one of the major ways your body removes acid from itself), let it sit around for a while and you'll be surprised how healthy (I'm sorry alkaline) your urine becomes. Additionally, if a "medical doctor" wants to know your acid-base status, we check your blood, not your urine.

Finally, we've gotten you back to a common sense approach; you know, where your grandparents were before we confused them and you. It's time to take a look at some of the specific problems we're confronted with today. Namely, how to eat out without dying out, how to improve what you're eating without wishing you were dead, and what to make for holiday meals without gaining 7 to 10 pounds in the process.

Figure 1. BALANCE NOT EXTREMISM IS THE KEY.

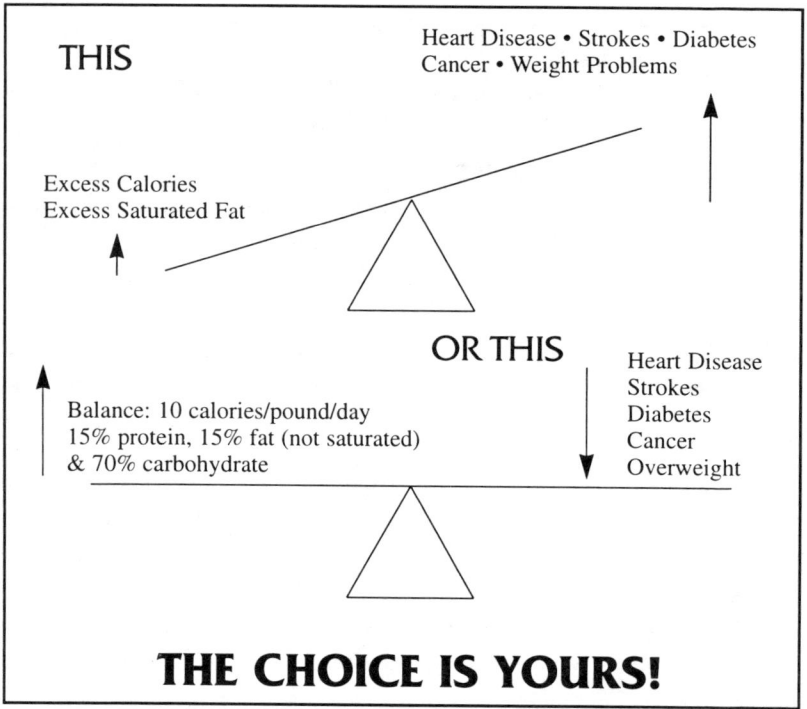

Chapter Nine.
One Thing About Fast food, *It's Fast.*

The American public has an insatiable appetite (yes this is a pun) for "fast food" restaurants. In fact in our fast-paced world, people want the quality of food they used to enjoy without the effort or time spent in preparing it. Restaurant managers and chefs have competed for our business by changing the flavor of the food they serve us. This is done primarily by adding fats, those same saturated fats we've been talking about since the beginning of this book.

One of the most frequently asked questions I hear when I'm giving a talk is what should you do when you eat out? The answer is to find out what the nutritional value of the food is you're planning to eat, and stick to your guidelines. All too often we go to restaurants and take what they give us. We seem to be more concerned with whether we're insulting them than we are with what we're eating. The truth is, we're paying for the food and it should meet our expectations. We shouldn't be meeting the restaurants expectations. This is true for many things.

> **YOU SHOULD BE FUSSY ABOUT WHAT YOU EAT – YOU'RE PAYING FOR IT – IN MORE WAYS THAN ONE.**

I once heard a physician friend of mine (on public television) say that when looking for a hospital, look for one that could guarantee you treatment of a heart attack within 30 minutes of the time you walked into the Emergency Room. If the hospital couldn't guarantee that, find a different hospital. After all it's your life! I feel the same way about restaurants. If you can't get food prepared the way you want it or need it, or if you can't find out what the nutritional (see below) value of the food is – go elsewhere.

The same holds true for airlines and traveling. When I first presented the research on reversing heart disease and the role dietary habits played, I presented it in London at the Queen Elizabeth II Conference Center in the Fleming Room (Imagine That!). British Airways provided the meals enroute and imagine my surprise when the person scheduling the flight asked me if I wanted Western or Eastern Vegetarian for my meal. They not only had vegetarian meals, they had more than one type and they where rightfully proud of that. Many airlines can provide you with whatever type of meal you want or need, although you need to ask in advance. These meals have come a long way from where they started.

> **WHEN SCHEDULING AIRLINE FLIGHTS, ASK ABOUT SPECIAL MENUS IN ADVANCE. MOST AIRLINES ARE EAGER TO PLEASE THEIR CUSTOMERS.**

Everyone is in the habit of thinking they're invincible and physicians are certainly no exception. I know one doctor who, while vacationing in another country eating steak packaged in his home town, had a heart attack (cafe coronary) while eating the meat at a medical meeting. Talk about irony! Following this event, he changed his lifestyle and attempted to change everyone else's. If you're ready to improve what you're eating and interested in helping others (without beating them up), then read on. This is the part of the book you've been waiting for. In this chapter we will look at *"fast* (fat?) *food."*

While preparing this chapter, I did exactly what you would have to do if (except I calculated the percentages and eliminated the garbage) you wanted to figure out the nutritional value of the food you're eating at these restaurants. I walked up to the front counter, introduced myself (please use your name and not mine) and asked for any Nutritional Information they might have regarding their food. I went to pizza places, hamburger shops, Italian, Japanese, Chinese, and Vietnamese Restaurants. I even went to Jennie Craig.

The vast majority of people said they didn't have anything but wanted me to know their food was "low fat," or they'd be glad to have corporate (headquarters) send me something. I didn't think this was very practical since you don't have time to wait for corporate to get back to you while you're waiting in line to eat, and this book isn't an ad for those restaurants. You know, I can go to the library and learn how to build a bomb, but getting nutritional information out of some of these people has got to be more difficult than getting Government secrets – no, I do not have any Government secrets. (I don't even have any good personal secrets.)

<u>NUTRITIONAL INFORMATION
– THE FAST FOOD INDUSTRY –
IN "ALPHABETICAL ORDER"</u>

The first "fast food" establishment to provide information had one of the best guides I've seen. They not only listed the nutrients of the foods, but they talked about food allergies and the ingredients of each of its foods. There were some inconsistencies in all of the nutritional guidelines provided, but in general the information was relatively complete. This is a great place to point out that I have no stock in any of these companies, so there is no problem with financial conflicts and my objective reporting of the numbers below. The only way to stay sane, and educate while writing, is to keep clean of these "conflicts of interest."

While many of these guidelines include information about vitamins, these aren't the foods you're buying for vitamins, so we are going to stay with the important issues of serving size, calories, total fat (grams/gm & percent of total calories/%), saturated fat (grams/gm & percent of total fat/%), carbohydrates (grams/gm & percent of total calories/%) and protein (grams/gm & percent of total calories) so you can compare these foods with the recommendations made in this book. None of the nutritional materials reported the percent of calories from protein or carbohydrate, emphasizing the obsession with percent fat calories, but missing the more important overall issue of balance.

> **MOST NUTRITIONAL LABELS ARE MISSING THE MOST IMPORTANT PIECES OF INFORMATION.**

Also at the request of many of my patients and people I have talked with, I am including sodium (milligrams/mg) in the tables. I am not including the cholesterol content, because it is the percent saturated fat and the overall calories which are the primary determinants of cholesterol levels in the blood, and I do not wish to have the reader led astray by extraneous information.

ARBY'S

Food	Serving	Calories	Total Fat	Sat Fat	Carb	Protein	Sodium
Bacon	two strips	90	7 (7%)	3 (43%)	0 (0%)	5 (30%)	220
Plain Biscuit	one	280	15 (48%)	3 (20%)	34 (49%)	2 (3%)	730
Blueberry muffin	one	230	9 (35%)	2 (22%)	35 (61%)	2 (4%)	290
Cinnamon nut danish	one	360	11 (27%)	1 (9%)	60 (67%)	6 (6%)	105
Croissant (plain)	one	220	12 (49%)	7 (58%)	25 (45%)	4 (6%)	230
Egg portion	one portion	95	8 (76%)	2 (25%)	0.5 (2%)	0.5 (2%)	54
French Toastix	six pieces	430	21 (44%)	5 (24%)	55 (51%)	5 (5%)	550
Ham	one	45	2 (38%)	0.5 (50%)	0 (0%)	7 (62%)	405
Sausage	one	163	15 (83%)	6 (40%)	0 (0%)	7 (17%)	321
Swiss	one	45	3 (60%)	2 (67%)	0.5 (4%)	4 (36%)	175

ARBY'S, cont.

Food	Serving	Calories	Total Fat	Sat Fat	Carb	Protein	Sodium
Table Syrup	one ounce	100	0 (0%)	0 (0%)	25 (100%)	0 (0%)	30
Arby's Melt with Cheddar	one	368	18 (43%)	6 (33%)	38 (41%)	18 (16%)	937
Bac'n Cheddar Deluxe	one	539	34 (57%)	10 (29%)	41 (30%)	22 (13%)	1140
Giant Roast Beef	one	555	28 (45%)	11 (39%)	48 (35%)	35 (20%)	1561
Regular Roast Beef	one	388	19 (44%)	7 (37%)	36 (37%)	23 (19%)	1009
Breaded Chicken Filet	one	536	28 (46%)	5 (18%)	51 (38%)	28 (16%)	1016
Chicken Cordon Bleu	one	623	33 (47%)	8 (24%)	51 (33%)	38 (20%)	1594
Chicken Fingers	two	290	16 (50%)	2 (12%)	20 (28%)	16 (22%)	677
French Dip Sandwich	one	475	22 (41%)	8 (36%)	43 (36%)	30 (23%)	1411
Hot Ham'n Swiss	one	500	23 (41%)	7 (30%)	45 (36%)	30 (23%)	1664
Light Roast Beef Deluxe	one	296	10 (30%)	3 (30%)	39 (53%)	18 (17%)	826
Light Roast Chicken Deluxe	one	276	6 (22%)	2 (33%)	37 (54%)	20 (24%)	777
Light Roast Turkey Deluxe	one	260	7 (21%)	2 (28%)	37 (57%)	20 (22%)	1262
Fish Fillet	one	529	27 (46%)	7 (26%)	52 (39%)	23 (15%)	864
Cheddar Curley Fries	3-1/2 ounces	333	18 (49%)	4 (22%)	40 (48%)	5 (3%)	1016
Homestyle Fries	"small"	212	10 (41%)	2 (20%)	31 (58%)	2.5 (1%)	414
Baked Potato (Plain)	11-1/2 ounce	384	0.3 (0%)	0 (0%)	89 (90%)	7 (10%)	26

One of the biggest surprises isn't the amount of fat or even saturated fat present in these foods, but the overall calories in one serving and the amount of salt present. The only truly healthy food here is the plain baked potato, that won't be so healthy for you after adding all the toppings they ask you if you want. The other thing worth pointing out is the fat and calories present in the fish fillet. Most people think that ordering chicken or fish will reduce the calories and fat present. This is true until you consider how the chicken or fish is coated and cooked. Frying in oil (100% fat) isn't a healthy approach to cooking and it's only going to increase the calories and fat eaten.

> **THE UNHEALTHIEST THING ABOUT THE FOOD WE EAT IS WHAT WE DO TO IT.**

BURGER KING

In the following table I have included shakes. At the end of this section I have include a table on "soft-drinks," given the popularity of these and the number of calories they have.

Food	Serving	Calories	Total Fat	Sat Fat	Carb	Protein	Sodium
Morning Biscuit Croissan' wich (with egg, sausage & cheese)	one	330	18 (48%)	4 (22%)	40 (48%)	6 (4%)	950
	one	550	42 (69%)	14 (33%)	27 (19%)	20 (12%)	1110
Hash Browns	small	240	15 (58%)	6 (40%)	27 (39%)	2 (3%)	440
Hamburger	one	330	15 (42%)	6 (40%)	33 (40%)	20 (18%)	530
Cheese-burger	one	380	19 (45%)	9 (47%)	34 (36%)	23 (19%)	770
Double cheese-burger with bacon	one	640	39 (55%)	18 (46%)	34 (21%)	44 (24%)	1240

BURGER KING, cont.

Food	Serving	Calories	Total Fat	Sat Fat	Carb	Protein	Sodium
Whopper Double	one	640	39 (55%)	11 (28%)	56 (35%)	27 (10%)	870
Whopper	one	870	56 (57%)	19 (34%)	56 (26%)	46 (17%)	940
BK Big Fish	one	720	43 (54%)	9 (21%)	66 (37%)	23 (9%)	1180
BK Broiler Chicken	one	530	26 (43%)	5 (19%)	52 (39%)	29 (18%)	1060
Broiled Chicken Salad	one	190	8 (37%)	4 (50%)	17 (30%)	20 (33%)	500
French Fries	medium	400	21 (48%)	8 (38%)	54 (51%)	3 (1%)	820
Onion Rings	one order	310	14 (42%)	2 (14%)	53 (51%)	4 (7%)	810
Vanilla shake	medium	300	6 (17%)	4 (67%)	53 (71%)	9 (12%)	230
Chocolate shake	medium	320	7 (18%)	4 (57%)	54 (67%)	9 (15%)	230
Chocolate shake (syrup added)	medium	440	7 (14%)	4 (57%)	84 (76%)	10 (10%)	430
Strawberry shake (syrup added)	medium	420	6 (12%)	4 (67%)	83 (79%)	9 (9%)	260

BRUEGGER'S BAGELS

Bagels have become a rather popular food in recent years, although the amount of fat ranges from 1 to 4 grams. Those listed below range from 1.5 to 2.5 grams without the extras. Like most food, it's what you add to it or how you prepare something (bake, fry, et cetera) that determines whether it's good for you or not. Most of the bagel spreads are extremely high in fat, even the "light" versions. We have also included various meats and fillers (hummus and tuna salad) used on bagels. An interesting trend in some restaurants

THE DIET MYTH

is the addition of a variety of "healthier" (not necessarily "healthy") foods, eg. soups, which do tend to be better for you, although the salt content could be a problem. You also shouldn't assume that just because something sounds like it's good for you doesn't mean it is.

Food	Serving	Calories	Total Fat	Sat Fat	Carb	Protein	Sodium
Roast Beef	one slice	70	1.5 (21%)	1 (67%)	0 (0%)	13 (79%)	580
Roasted Turkey	one slice	60	0.5 (8%)	0 (0%)	0 (0%)	13 (92%)	580
Smoked Turkey	one slice	70	0.5 (7%)	0 (0%)	2 (11%)	15 (82%)	760
Ham	one slice	80	2.5 (31%)	1 (40%)	3 (15%)	12 (54%)	820
Hummus	one	150	9 (53%)	1.5 (17%)	13 (35%)	5 (12%)	140
Tuna Salad	one	260	19 (65%)	3 (16%)	9 (14%)	12 (21%)	580
Chicken Salad	one	190	8 (37%)	2 (25%)	5 (10%)	24 (53%)	555
	B	A	G	E	L	S	
Cinnamon Raisin	one	290	1.5 (3%)	0 (0%)	60 (83%)	10 (14%)	400
Plain	one	280	1.5 (5%)	0 (0%)	56 (80%)	10 (15%)	430
Blueberry	one	300	2 (7%)	0 (0%)	60 (80%)	10 (13%)	480
Poppy Seed	one	280	1.5 (5%)	0 (0%)	57 (81%)	11 (14%)	440
Sundried Tomato	one	280	1.5 (5%)	0 (0%)	56 (80%)	10 (15%)	490
Sesame	one	290	2.5 (7%)	0.5 (20%)	57 (79%)	11 (14%)	440
Garlic	one	280	1.5 (4%)	0 (%)	57 (81%)	10 (15%)	440
Onion	one	280	1.5 (4%)	0 (0%)	57 (81%)	10 (15%)	430
Honey Grain	one	300	2.5 (8%)	0.5 (20%)	58 (77%)	11 (15%)	390
Everything	one	290	2 (7%)	0 (0%)	58 (80%)	11 (13%)	700
	S	O	U	P	S		
Aztec Chicken	8 ounces	100	3 (30%)	0.5 (17%)	11 (44%)	7 (26%)	1020
Big Chili	8 ounces	230	11 (39%)	4 (36%)	20 (35%)	17 (26%)	1130
Black Bean	8 ounces	110	2 (14%)	0 (0%)	18 (65%)	5 (21%)	660
Cajun Gumbo	8 ounces	80	0 (0%)	0 (0%)	16 (80%)	3 (20%)	440
Clam Chowder	8 ounces	180	9 (44%)	5 (55%)	19 (42%)	9 (14%)	990
Minestrone	8 ounces	70	0.5 (7%)	0 (0%)	15 (86%)	3 (7%)	850
Turkey Orzo	8 ounces	80	15 (19%)	0 (0%)	7 (35%)	9 (46%)	920

DAIRY QUEEN

How healthy are those snacks we're eating? While you're probably going to be disappointed (not surprised, just disappointed), I thought I should include these because I've always thought if we could get all the world leaders to sit down around a bowel of ice-cream (frozen yogurt/sorbet), this world would be a safer, more peaceful place to live. Have you ever seen anyone angry while they were eating ice-cream?

Food	Serving	Calories	Total Fat	Sat Fat	Carb	Protein	Sodium
Vanilla Soft Serve	1/2 cup	140	4.5 (28%)	3 (67%)	22 (62%)	3 (12%)	70
Vanilla Cone	medium	330	9 (27%)	6 (67%)	53 (64%)	8 (9%)	160
Nonfat Frozen Yogurt	1/2 cup	100	0 (0%)	0 (0%)	21 (84%)	3 (16%)	70
Yogurt Cone	medium	260	1 (4%)	0.5 (50%)	56 (86%)	9 (10%)	160
Chocolate Malt	medium	880	22 (23%)	14 (64%)	153 (70%)	19 (7%)	500
Chocolate Shake	medium	770	20 (23%)	13 (65%)	130 (68%)	17 (9%)	420
Chocolate Sundae	small	280	7 (21%)	4.5 (64%)	49 (70%)	5 (9%)	140
Chocolate Sundae	medium	400	10 (22%)	6 (60%)	71 (71%)	8 (7%)	210
Banana Split	one	510	12 (20%)	8 (67%)	96 (75%)	8 (5%)	180
Peanut Buster Parfait	one	730	31 (38%)	17 (55%)	99 (54%)	16 (8%)	400
Chocolate Chip Cookie Blizzard	medium	950	36 (34%)	19 (53%)	143 (60%)	17 (6%)	660

A lot of what we've been talking about in this book is using common sense. Is it any wonder why so many Americans are overweight (including one-third of our children) when many of the foods we eat have more calories and fat than many people throughout the world would eat in an entire day?

THE DIET MYTH

One of the marketing tools used by many restaurants, is the heart healthy symbol, or a heart, beside an item on the menu. I've listened to many people justify these not-so-heart-healthy food selections by saying that if a person eats a sensible diet in addition to the items identified as "heart healthy," that the entire diet will fit with the heart-healthy scheme of things. This however, doesn't make the "heart healthy" item truly "heart healthy." It just means that everything else you eat is making up for it. This is similar to the herbal remedies which say if you use their product, in addition to a heart-healthy diet, you'll see a lowering of your cholesterol level. By the way, you'll see the same lowering of your cholesterol by following the "heart-healthy diet" without the herbal (vitamin, or whatever) product, without having to pay for something you really don't need or benefit from.

FERNANDO'S

Many restaurants, like the next one have information about calories and fat, but nothing about carbohydrates or protein. This shows our fascination with calories (since 1915), but our failure to recognize the importance of "saturated fat," and our failure to look at the overall balance of calories, fats, carbohydrates and protein in our diet. Nonetheless, the following "Mexican Restaurant" had some information from 1995, which was better than what most of the restaurants had.

Food	Calories	Total Fat	Sodium
Chicken Taco	238	8 (30%)	538
Deluxe Taco	361	12 (30%)	709
Chicken Enchilada	327	10 (28%)	1042
Bean Burrito	489	10 (18%)	1080
Bean Tostada	318	7 (20%)	382
Seafood Enchilada	369	12 (29%)	554
Fajita Salad	401	12 (27%)	497
Grilled Chicken Sandwich with Rice and Salad	539	12 (20%)	679

RICHARD M. FLEMING, M.D.

> **GOOD TASTE DOESN'T MEAN IT HAS TO BE BAD FOR YOU.**

The trend that I find interesting for the foods listed here is the lower-than-expected percentage of fat in each of these recipes. While these are probably the recipes they are most proud of (and rightfully so), they clearly demonstrate that food which tastes good, doesn't have to be bad for you.

GARDEN CAFE & BAKERY

The following is an example of overusing the word "heart." While I'm glad to see an interest in healthy eating, the use of the word "heart" or "heart healthy" has a wide range of meaning as shown by the wide range in calories (227-512), total fat (5-32%) – who knows how much is "saturated fat," and sodium (salt) which ranged from 408-884 milligrams per serving.

Food	Calories	Total Fat	Sodium
Heart French Toast with low Calorie Syrup	368	3 (7%)	571
Heart French Toast with Applesauce	324	3 (8%)	459
Heart Omelette with Fruit	227	2 (8%)	443
Heart Omelette with Bran Muffin	405	12 (27%)	864
Heart Omelette with Low Fat Muffin	375	2 (5%)	884
Heart Chicken Filet Sandwich with Fresh Fruit	512	16 (28%)	408
Heart Melt with Fresh Fruit	330	10 (27%)	743
Bran Muffin	280	10 (32%)	440

GODFATHER'S PIZZA

Pizza is an example of a change in the American Diet that occurred over the last several decades. It is also an example of something we can do wrong <u>or right</u>. Many people are not aware that there are relatively sophisticated computer (software) programs available which will give the nutritional information on most of the foods we have or can make. This information can be used to improve the quality and flavor of the food we eat. The following examples show how simple differences in the dough and toppings used for a pizza can result in major changes in the nutritional value of the pizza. For example, dough made with oil added (Golden Crust) versus dough made without added oil (Original Crust) are significantly different in calories, percent of fat, carbohydrates and protein. Even the amount of salt is different. The same technique of using no-stick cooking sprays can be used in your home. Unfortunately the "saturated fat" information was not available (NA).

Food	Serving	Calories	Total Fat	Sat Fat	Carb	Protein	Sodium
O	R	I	G	I	N	A	L
Cheese (MINI)	1/4 Pizza	131	3 (21%)	NA	19 (58%)	7 (21%)	183
Cheese (Medium)	1/8 Pizza	231	5 (19%)	NA	34 (59%)	13 (22%)	338
Cheese (Large)	1/10 Pizza	258	6 (21%)	NA	36 (56%)	15 (23%)	396
Cheese (Jumbo)	1/10 Pizza	382	9 (21%)	NA	53 (55%)	22 (24%)	580
Comb (Mini)	1/4 Pizza	176	7 (36%)	NA	21 (48%)	10 (16%)	382
Combo (Medium)	1/8 Pizza	306	11 (32%)	NA	36 (47%)	17 (21%)	660
Combo (Large)	1/10 Pizza	338	12 (32%)	NA	38 (45%)	19 (23%)	740
Combo (Jumbo)	1/10 Pizza	503	18 (32%)	NA	56 (45%)	29 (23%)	1096
		G	O	L	D	E	N
Cheese (Medium)	1/8 Pizza	212	8 (34%)	NA	26 (49%)	10 (17%)	311

GODFATHER'S PIZZA, cont.

Food	Serving	Calories	Total Fat	Sat Fat	Carb	Protein	Sodium
Cheese (Large)	1/10 Pizza	242	9 (33%)	NA	28 (46%)	12 (21%)	363
Combo (Medium)	1/8 Pizza	271	12 (40%)	NA	28 (41%)	13 (19%)	562
Combo (Large)	1/10 Pizza	305	14 (41%)	NA	31 (41%)	16 (18%)	674

As you can see from the pizza examples shown above, the higher the percent fat present, the lower the percent of protein. A good rule of thumb when eating out, is to assume that if the percent of calories from fat in something you're going to eat increases, the percent of calories from protein will be going down.

For decades we have been promoting, or at least talking about, healthier eating habits. We have been confusing many people by talking about all this as "changing your diet," thereby allowing the "diet" industry to capitalize on the theme of "dieting." This has the potential of promoting many unhealthy and dangerous "dietary" practices, and the exploitation/selling of vitamins, herbs and supplements by "healthcare practitioners" and others who are looking to make a profit from all this confusion. Many of these people believe they are "qualified" to provide nutritional advice when they're really not. Only by educating the general public and overcoming these misconceptions can we hope to promote sound nutritional change within the United States and Western society, and among the different cultures within our society.

McDONALD'S

Several months ago a friend told me the story he had heard about why McDonald's (many years ago) decided to change from frying their french-fries in beef talo to vegetable oil. As the story goes, one person took it upon himself to advertise on radio about how frying french fries in vegetable oil instead of beef talo, would reduce the amount of saturated fat in McDonalds french fries and subsequently

THE DIET MYTH

reduce the health risk to the people who were eating McDonalds french fries. The advertising worked and not only did McDonalds change to vegetable oil (with less saturated fat), but so did its competitors.

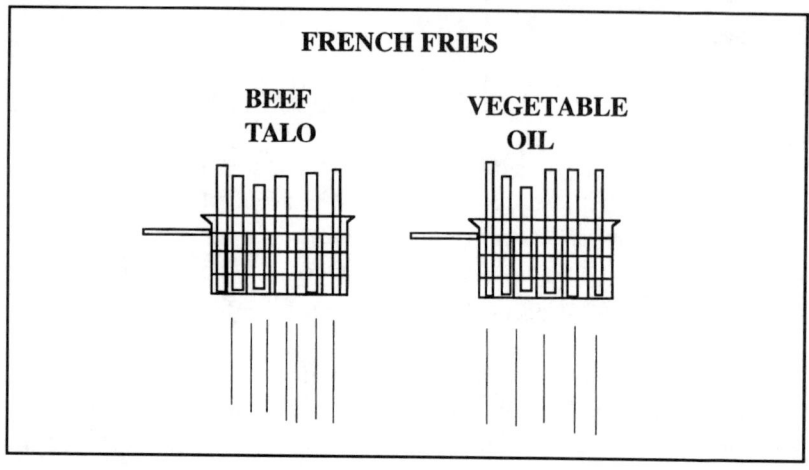

Food	Serving	Calories	Total Fat	Sat Fat	Carb	Protein	Sodium
Egg McMuffin	one	290	12 (38%)	4.5 (38%)	27 (37%)	17 (25%)	710
Sausage McMuffin	one	360	23 (58%)	8 (35%)	26 (29%)	13 (13%)	740
English Muffin	one	140	2 (14%)	0 (0%)	25 (71%)	4 (15%)	210
Sausage	one order	170	16 (88%)	5 (31%)	0 (0%)	6 (12%)	290
Scrambled Eggs	two	160	11 (62%)	3.5 (32%)	1 (2%)	13 (36%)	170
Hash Browns	one order	130	8 (54%)	1.5 (19%)	14 (43%)	1 (3%)	330
Pancakes	one order	310	7 (19%)	1.5 (21%)	53 (68%)	9 (13%)	610
Pancakes with 2 pats of margarine and syrup	one order	580	16 (26%)	3 (19%)	100 (69%)	9 (5%)	760
Breakfast Burrito	one	320	20 (56%)	7 (35%)	23 (29%)	13 (15%)	600

The average egg may have anywhere between 215 and 425 milligrams (mgs) of cholesterol (remember we're trying to keep cholesterol intake down to 200 to 300 mgs per day). The biggest problem with eggs is the amount of fat (particularly saturated fat) they have. In the above example, we can see that 62% of the total calories are fat with 32% of the fat calories being "saturated." Some efforts are being taken to change the fat in eggs, by changing what the chickens are eating to include a greater amount of "polyunsaturated" fats, much like we're trying to get you to do when you eat (ie. exchange the saturated fat for polyunsaturated fat). The result appears to be similar for chickens and people. For chickens, the eggs appear to end up with more of the essential omega-3 fatty acids we need (as we discussed in chapter 3) and less of the "saturated" fats we don't need.

McDONALD'S (cont.)

Food	Serving	Calories	Total Fat	Sat Fat	Carb	Protein	Sodium
Hamburger	one	260	9 (31%)	3.5 (39%)	34 (52%)	13 (17%)	580
Cheeseburger	one	320	13 (38%)	6 (46%)	35 (44%)	15 (18%)	820
Quarter Pounder	one	420	21 (45%)	8 (38%)	37 (35%)	23 (20%)	820
Big Mac	one	560	31 (50%)	10 (32%)	45 (32%)	26 (18%)	1070
Crispy Chick Deluxe	one	500	25 (44%)	4 (16%)	43 (34%)	26 (22%)	1100
Fish Fillet Deluxe	one	560	28 (45%)	6 (21%)	54 (39%)	23 (16%)	1060
Grilled Chick Fillet	one	440	20 (41%)	3 (15%)	38 (34%)	27 (25%)	1040
French Fries	small	210	10 (43%)	1.5 (15%)	26 (50%)	3 (7%)	135
French Fries	large	450	22 (44%)	4 (18%)	57 (50%)	6 (6%)	290
French Fries	Super size	540	26 (43%)	4.5 (17%)	68 (50%)	8 (7%)	350
Chicken McNuggets	9 pieces	430	26 (53%)	5 (19%)	23 (21%)	27 (26%)	770
Hot Mustard	one pkg.	60	3.5 (50%)	0 (0%)	7 (47%)	1 (3%)	240
Sweet 'N Sour Sauce	one pkg.	50	0 (0%)	0 (0%)	11 (100%)	0 (0%)	140
Light Mayonnaise	one pkg.	40	4 (90%)	0.5 (1%)	1 (10%)	0 (0%)	85
Grilled Chick Salad Deluxe	one	120	1.5 (8%)	0 (0%)	7 (23%)	21 (69%)	240

THE DIET MYTH

Once again we are reminded that the way we cook or prepare food is the important key to understanding how much fat, particularly saturated fat, we will be eating. The grilled chicken salad is not only low in calories, but has no saturated fat and is "filling." Another problem is the number of calories and the amount of fat (particularly saturated fat) we add to our food simply by adding salad dressings and "sauces." The "Light Mayonnaise" used on the above sandwiches is ninety percent fat and adds nothing to the value of the food we're eating.

The following selection is from an "Italian" restaurant chain.

THE OLIVE GARDEN

Food	Serving	Calories	Total Fat	Sat Fat	Carb	Protein	Sodium
Capellini Pomodoro	12 ounces	380	10 (23%)	2 (20%)	60 (69%)	13 (8%)	1030
Capellini Primavera	12 ounces	350	7 (19%)	3 (43%)	58 (66%)	14 (15%)	820
Capellini Primavera with Chicken	16 ounces	510	13 (23%)	4.5 (35%)	59 (46%)	39 (31%)	1550
Chicken Giardino	13 ounces	360	9 (22%)	3.5 (39%)	47 (52%)	23 (26%)	900
Linguine alla Marinara	19.5 ounces	330	6 (17%)	0.5 (8%)	57 (69%)	10 (14%)	710
Shrimp Primavera	15-3/4 ounces	400	6 (14%)	2.5 (42%)	61 (61%)	26 (25%)	820
Grilled Chicken Capri	21 ounces	550	12 (19%)	3.5 (29%)	52 (38%)	58 (43%)	1660
Apple Caramellina	12 ounces	560	2 (3%)	1 (50%)	131 (94%)	6 (3%)	190

These particular selections demonstrate how meats and pastas can be combined to make complete entrees (main courses). This is typical of the traditional Mediterranean approach to eating where heart disease is less of a problem. One of the major differences between sauces/toppings added to pastas is the difference between "white sauces" which are cream/milk based (with plenty of additional calories and fat) and marinara sauces which are tomato based. The Linguine alla Marinara in the table above has only 330 calories (19.5 ounces is 1.2 pounds of food), and it has an almost ideal proportion of fats, carbohydrates and proteins.

What I was particularly impressed by with the next restaurant establishment was that despite only having one copy of their nutritional information sheet, they went and photocopied what they had so I could have a copy to take with me. Hopefully, your service will be just as pleasant.

SUBWAY

Food	Serving	Calories	Total Fat	Sodium
Veggie Delite	6 inch sub	223	3 (12%)	526
Turkey Breast	6 inch sub	276	4 (13%)	1303
Turkey Breast and Ham	6 inch sub	275	4 (13%)	1297
Ham	6 inch sub	273	4 (13%)	1291
Roast Beef	6 inch sub	299	6 (18%)	837
Subway Club	6 inch sub	300	6 (18%)	1261
Seafood and Crab	6 inch sub	415	19 (41%)	793
Cold Cut Trio	6 inch sub	347	12 (31%)	1222
Tuna	6 inch sub	522	33 (57%)	824
Roasted Chicken Breast Fillet	6 inch sub	321	5 (14%)	1065
Steak & Cheese	6 inch sub	363	10 (25%)	1079
Subway Melt	6 inch sub	361	12 (30%)	1680
Meatball	6 inch sub	411	15 (33%)	1014

Like most of the food we've seen so far, there is a wide variety in what's available at any given restaurant, with some foods having the right amount of total fat. Unfortunately there is no information available about saturated fat, carbohydrate or protein content at this restaurant.

THE DIET MYTH

The last food chain is familiar to many people. It did at one time have a salad line which has since been discontinued. The critics were right, you don't go to "fast food" restaurants to eat salads. TOO BAD!

WENDY'S

One important piece of information to consider when reading the following table is that each of the food items is separate. If you are having a bun with your hamburger (most people do) you have to add these two numbers together. You also need to remember to add all the toppings/condiments (eg. ketchup, mustard, pickles, et cetera) for your final calorie, fat, carbohydrate and protein counts. This includes the Pita dressings as well. While we will not include a list of the condiments here, don't assume these are free of calories, fat or anything else. When you add a single piece of American Cheese you're adding 70 calories, fifty of which (71%) are fat calories. Of these, 31 (63%) are saturated fat. There are also 320 milligrams of sodium in this one slice of cheese.

Food	Serving	Calories	Total Fat	Sat Fat	Carb	Protein	Sodium
Hamburger	1/4 pound	200	14 (60%)	6 (43%)	0 (0%)	19 (40%)	290
Grilled Chick Fillet	one piece	110	3 (23%)	1 (33%)	0 (0%)	22 (77%)	450
Breaded Chick Fillet	one piece	230	12 (43%)	2.5 (21%)	10 (17%)	22 (40%)	490
Spicy Chick Fillet	one piece	210	9 (38%)	1.5 (17%)	10 (19%)	22 (57%)	920
Kaiser Bun	one	190	3 (16%)	0.5 (17%)	36 (76%)	6 (8%)	340
Sandwich Bun	one	160	2.5 (16%)	0.5 (20%)	29 (72%)	5 (12%)	280
Chicken Caesar Pita	one	490	18 (33%)	5 (28%)	48 (39%)	34 (28%)	1320
Classic Greek Pita	one	440	20 (41%)	8 (20%)	50 (45%)	15 (14%)	1050
Garden Ranch Chick Pita	one	480	18 (33%)	4 (22%)	51 (42%)	30 (25%)	1180
Garden Veggie Pita	one	400	17 (38%)	3.5 (20%)	52 (52%)	11 (10%)	760

This last example is classic for how "veggie" has been used as a marketing tool to get you (the consumer) to assume that something is "good" for you or "better" than something which doesn't have "veggie" attached to it, and why "vegetarian" diets don't necessarily work. Vegetarian recipes are notorious for having relatively high amounts of fats present, without the meat. In the example above, the Garden Veggie Pita has the same number of fat grams (17 versus 18) as the Chicken Caesar and Garden Ranch Pitas, which aren't vegetarian. The only thing less is the protein.

Before leaving this section we should briefly touch on something typically forgotten by people when counting calories. That is, namely, the soft-drinks (pop, soda, et cetera) that have become such a part of our society. Schools have added vending machines to their school lunch rooms (and elsewhere) because students "want" the pop. This is a very interesting argument, since it in no way implies that the pop is good or even necessary for the children. The argument that they "want" the pop could be used to put beer, alcohol and cigarette machines in the school, because it's no secret, many of the students want these too. We wouldn't do it of course, WHY? Because we know that these aren't healthy for our children.

So why are we allowing students access to these other vending (pop, candy, et cetera) machines. I've had teachers tell me that students can't afford to buy school lunches because the money they bring with them from home is spent on vending machines, and all too often the parents aren't aware of where the money is going. Soft-drinks are not the root of the problems in schools, but there truly is not a need for them in the schools, particularly when 25-35% of all students from K-12th grade are overweight, have diabetes, high blood pressure, or have high cholesterol levels. The habits they build today will be the ones they live or die with tomorrow.

> **WE WOULDN'T DREAM OF LETTING STUDENTS HAVE CIGARETTE OR ALCOHOL MACHINES AT SCHOOL.**

THE DIET MYTH

The following is meant to be a partial list of soft-drinks and it doesn't adequately address the issue of **caffeine** because the amount of caffeine per serving is no longer listed (out of sight, out of mind). All of the calories present in soft-drinks are from sugars, none come from fats or proteins. Finally, artificial sweeteners in diet pops need to be addressed since they are a real concern to many people who are unable to handle (phenyl<u>ketonuria</u>) the amino acid Phenylalanine. Note that the ending of this genetic abnormality includes the term "<u>ketonuria</u>." This term, which means the addition of ketone acids to the urine, was the same concern we talked about earlier for people who were eating high-protein, low-carbohydrate "diets" as promoted by many popular, but alarming books. When this problem occurs in the diabetic individual, "Medical Doctors" take it seriously and we call it <u>d</u>iabetic (DKA) <u>k</u>et<u>oa</u>cidosis.

SOFT (?) - DRINKS

Soft-Drink	Serving	Calories	Carbo-hydrates (grams)	Sodium	Caffeine Present	Phenyl-alanine Present
A & W Root Beer	12 oz	170	46	45	No	No
Diet A & W Root Beer	12 oz	0	0	0	No	Yes
A & W Cream Soda	12 oz	180	46	45	Yes	No
Diet A & W Cream Soda	12 oz	0	0	70	Yes	Yes
Barq's Root Beer	12 oz	160	45	70	Yes	No
Canada Dry (Ginger Ale)	12 oz	120	33	40	No	No
Clearly Canadian (Raspberry Cream)	11 oz	100	26	15	No	No
Clearly Canadian (Fruit & Berries, Wild Cherry)	11 oz	120	31	15	No	No
Clearly Canadian (Fraire-Melon, Peach Mango)	11 oz	110	27	15	No	No
Clearly Canadian (Blackberry)	11 oz	130	32	15	No	No
Coke	12 oz	140	39	39	Yes	No
Diet Coke	12 oz	0	0	40	Yes	Yes

SOFT (?) - DRINKS, cont.

Soft-Drink	Serving	Calories	Carbo-hydrates (grams)	Sodium	Caffeine Present	Phenyl-alanine Present
Classic Coke	12 oz	140	39	50	Yes	No
Caffeine Free Classic Coke	12 oz	140	39	50	No	No
Diet Rite Cola	12 oz	0	0	0	No	Yes
Dr. Pepper	12 oz	150	40	55	Yes	No
Caffeine Free Dr. Pepper	12 oz	150	40	55	No	No
Diet Dr. Pepper	12 oz	0	0	55	Yes	Yes
Diet - Caffeine Free Dr. Pepper	12 oz	0	0	55	No	Yes
Fresca	12 oz	0	0	35	No	Yes
Kick	12 oz	180	49	50	Yes	No
Mr. Pibb	12 oz	140	39	45	Yes	No
Mountain Dew	12 oz	165	46	75	Yes	No
Diet Mountain Dew	12 oz	0	0	0	Yes	Yes
Mug Root Beer	12 oz	160	43	65	No	No
Diet Mug Root Beer	12 oz	0	0	0	No	Yes
Pepsi	12 oz	150	41	35	Yes	No
Pepsi without caffeine	12 oz	150	41	35	No	No
Diet Pepsi	12 oz	0	0	0	Yes	Yes
Wild Cherry Pepsi	12 oz	160	43	35	Yes	No
Royal Crown Cola	12 oz	150	42	50	Yes	No
Schweppes (Ginger Ale)	12 oz	130	33	75	No	No
7-Up	12 oz	140	39	75	No	No
Diet 7-Up	12 oz	0	0	35	No	Yes
Cherry 7-Up	12 oz	140	39	35	No	No
Diet Cherry 7-Up	12 oz	0	0	35	No	Yes
Sioux City Sarsaparilla	12 oz	110	28	30	No	No
Sioux City Cream Soda	12 oz	180	45	30	No	No
Slice (Lemon-Lime)	12 oz	150	39	52	No	No
Slice (Orange)	12 oz	165	46	52	Yes	No
Dr. Slice	12 oz	140	39	35	Yes	No
Sprite	12 oz	140	38	70	No	No
Squirt	12 oz	150	40	25	No	No
Surge	12 oz	180	46	38	Yes	No
Vernors (Ginger Soda)	12 oz	150	39	25	No	No
Diet Vernors (Ginger Soda)	12 oz	0	0	25	No	Yes

THE DIET MYTH

Modern conveniences have made our lives so much easier than the lives of our parents and grandparents, but some of that has come with a price. Whether we're driving all day (instead of walking), or buying food at a restaurant that someone else has prepared (instead of us), we run the risk of not taking care of our bodies as well as we should. Simple differences like parking farther from where we want to walk, or being very choosy about the food we eat, can make a big difference.

Remember, you're going to pay someone to do something you can do for yourself, namely make a meal to eat. They're not paying you. You wouldn't dream of buying something you didn't want just because someone forced it on you, and you should be even more careful about what you eat when someone serves you food. As I mentioned in the first book *How to Bypass Your Bypass*, my great-grandparents started a restaurant chain in the Midwestern United States when my grandmother was just a girl. The importance of food has never been taken lightly in our family and it shouldn't be in yours. In the next chapter we're going to look at ways to improve the meals you're making at home. These include not only how to prepare the food, but how to cook it as well. Most of these approaches are very easy and reduce the overall calories and saturated fats in our diets, allowing us to continue to enjoy many of the foods we like and perhaps need in our diet.

Chapter Ten.
Improve your diet and enjoy what you're eating.

I'm always amazed when surveys are done looking at what foods (fruits, vegetables, et cetera) people like the most. They typically ask questions like "What fruit do you buy more of for your family?" They then compile the results and say, Americans rank the banana as the #1 fruit they like. What they seem to be missing is that while bananas are great for you, it doesn't mean that that's what people like most; it just happens to be less expensive to buy bananas right now than apples, oranges, grapes, plums; well, you get the picture. A problem for most of us seems to be where to spend the limited amount of money we have, as well as trying to figure out what's good for us.

> **WHAT WE'RE BUYING ISN'T NECESSARILY WHAT WE LIKE.**

Throughout this book we've emphasized the importance of reducing the number of calories and saturated fat currently present in our diet, while avoiding the gimmicky diets and programs designed to relieve you of that excess weight in your wallet. The problem with most prepackaged foods is that they are saturated (hydrogenated) so we can keep them on our pantry shelf without worrying about spoilage. They are also frequently less expensive. Foods which are not processed, typically not only are better for us, but taste better as well. Unfortunately they also tend to be more expensive, placing most of us in the uneasy position of trying to make ends meet financially while trying to feed our family and ourselves. Most of the time it feels like we're on a merry-go-round trying to make ends meet and satisfy our family's needs.

WHAT WE'RE BUYING ISN'T NECESSARILY GOOD FOR US.

Figure 1. The merry-go-round of preparing meals.

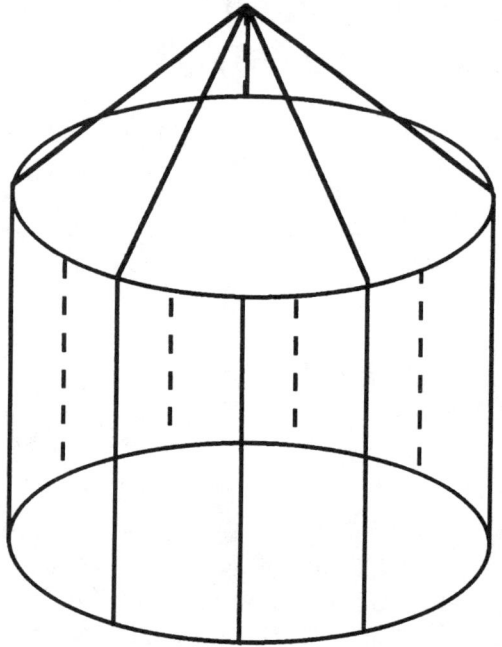

STARTING WITH THE BASICS

Most of us don't enjoy things that we consider drudgery. Many people look at preparing and eating food as either a chore or something they do in front of the television. The more rushed you are to make a meal and get it over with, the more likely you are to add unnecessary fats and calories to get the job over with as soon as possible. For most of us, we really don't need to rush through our meals, particularly during our evenings. This time of day, used to be spent talking about the days events and it provided the opportunity for families to socialize. While many people deny that need today, we have replaced it with going to restaurants with our "friends and family," where we eat and "socialize."

RICHARD M. FLEMING, M.D.

> **EATING AND SOCIALIZING GO HAND-IN-HAND, ESPECIALLY IF YOU HAVE CHILDREN.**

I also have to admit that it can be a lot of fun experimenting in the kitchen although I frequently don't know where many things are. My wife, from whom many of my really good ideas come, experiments constantly with different ways of cooking food without making it boring. The first thing you need to do IS TO TAKE A POSITIVE ATTITUDE while making meals.

The next thing you need to do is to decide what you're going to eat, not how you're going to prepare it. Decide whether you're planing to have meat, pasta, rice or something else as the main course (entree). This is the same thing you would do if you went out to eat. Once you've decided what you want to eat, you can then decide how to make it. Do you want to coat it with grease, lard, and fry it, or do you want to try something that doesn't cover up the flavor of what you're making, but improves it. If you're going to use a meat with skin on it (chicken, turkey, duck, et cetera), you can easily improve what you're going to eat by removing the skin. This removes calories, cholesterol and saturated fat, not to mention removing something we normally wouldn't eat if we thought about it. What if it doesn't have skin? The answer is obvious, we learned earlier that the saturated fat (the bad stuff) found in meat lies primarily in the fatty part. This includes beef, pork, lamb, veal, et cetera. Trimming away at least part of the fat will reduce some or most (depending on how much you trim) of the saturated fat and calories, and it's this part of the meat you shouldn't eat anyway. Fish has very little fat, if any, to remove. If you eat fish, you should remove the scales if it has scales.

> **IF IT HAS SKIN, REMOVE IT.
> IF IT HAS FAT, TRIM IT.**

Once you've removed the excess fats and calories by removing either the skin or trimming the fat, you can think about how you're going to cook it. When you add something to food, it ends up being absorbed by the food and then by you, so anything you add to the meat now should be something you think won't hurt you. A lot of people fry food because it's quick and easy. In reality there's not much difference in the amount of time it takes to fry, bake or grill most foods. Stir frying and broiling are quicker because stir frying cuts the meat into smaller pieces and broiling cooks from both directions.

The return of the convection oven has also helped reduce cooking time. If you don't think so, try cooking your next turkey in a convection oven. You won't need to be up at 6 am to start cooking. Baking, grilling and broiling are methods of dry cooking, which means no added oil is necessary to cook the meat, and the meat will cook in its own juices (oils). It's important to remember, that if the meat is sitting in the oil that comes out of it, the meat will simply reabsorb the fat. If you want to cook without additional oil and let the oils/fats from the meat drip out (the flavor will be even better), you should either grill the meat (oils drip away from the meat) or use a special broiling (or equivalent) pan to allow the meat to stand free of the juices.

> **BAKING, GRILLING & BROILING COOKS MEAT WITHOUT ADDED OIL.**

The flavor of meat can be enhanced by one of several methods. To begin with, meat can be marinated. This means you leave the meat sitting in a mixture of seasonings, herbs, et cetera and allow the meat the opportunity to absorb the flavor of the marinade sauce. This can be done by letting the meat sit in a bowel in the refrigerator immersed in the marinade during the day or overnight. It can be removed and cooked whenever you're ready for it. Table 1 shows some of the herbs and spices available today and what foods they can be used with.

Table 1. Herbs and Spices

Allspice	taste like blend of cinnamon cloves and nutmeg	for roasts, pea & tomato soup, squash and yams
Basil	member of the mint family and has slight licorice-like flavor and sweet smell	any tomato dish, fish, chicken, eggs, cottage cheese, zucchini, peas, carrots and salad dressings
Bay leaves	flavor mellows with cooking	soups, stews, spaghetti sauce, chili
Caraway seeds	slightly sharp taste	breads, sauerkraut, rice, cheese dishes, meat marinades
Celery seeds	flavor similar to celery but more intense	sauces, soups, meat, including fish, pickles and salads
Chili powder	to enhance hotness	Mexican-style dishes and chili con carne
Cinnamon	sweet and pungent flavor	Middle Eastern or Mediterranean style dishes
Cloves	sweet aroma and flavor	baked beans, green vegetables, spiced nuts, stewed fruits, cranberry relish
Coriander (or Cilantro)	stronger flavor than parsley, seeds are slightly citricy	salads, chili, tacos, enchiladas, stir fried vegetables
Dill	dill flavor	salmon, shellfish, tomatoes, carrots, cucumbers, potatoes
Fennel seeds	anise-like but not as sweet	macaroni or potato salad, lasagna, spaghetti or tomato soup
Ginger	sweet aroma, hot taste	vegetables, chicken or steak
Marjoram	similar to oregano	spaghetti, pizza, lasagna, stuffing for meats, salad and stewed tomatoes
Mint (peppermint & spearmint)	strong, sweet, cool	desserts, fruits & vegetables
Mustard	sharp, hot flavor	sauerkraut, potato salad, fish, crab, coleslaw
Nutmeg	sweet and spicy	meat loaf, eggnog, chicken, spinach and asparagus
Oregano	similar to marjoram but stronger	lamb, pork, beef, tomato and cheese dishes, vegetables
Paprika	mild and sweet, to hot with a bite	a garnish, also for veal & chicken

Parsley	parsley flavor	vegetables & fish
Pepper	black pepper	vegetables, meats, salads
Poppy seeds	nutty flavor	noodles, fruit salad, breads, pancakes
Red pepper	hot and pungent	tomato juice, Welsh rabbit, shrimp, crab, vegetable soup
Rosemary	bittersweet flavor	spaghetti, pizza, lasagna, lamb, pork and chicken, eggplant
Saffron	slightly bitter	Middle Eastern or Mediterranean style dishes
Sage	aromatic	turkey
Sesame seeds	nutlike flavor	vegetables, stuffed mushrooms, fruit salads and cottage cheese
Tarragon	anise like flavor	meats, salads, soups and stews
Thyme	lemon thyme has lemon flavor	vegetables, fish chowder, seafood, meats and tomato or cheese dishes
Turmeric	slightly bitter, musty flavor	chicken, seafood, pickles and relishes
Vanilla Bean	with age, a strong sweet flavor	for fruits, desserts and coffee

Like most foods, fresh is best and spices are no exception. Fresh herbs and red spices (paprika, chili pepper) should be refrigerated. Dried herbs along with ground or whole spices should be stored in a cool, dry, dark space. You don't have to be a master chef to realize that the spices and herbs shown above are just a few of many available. What we have discovered from other books is that frequently people just need a few ideas to get them started. The table above does just that. Once you've had the opportunity to experiment with some of these seasonings you will want to try others. There are several cookbooks available which you can use in conjunction with the recommendations from this book to allow you to cook truly healthy and tasty meals for you and your family/friends.

> **YOU DON'T HAVE TO BE A MASTER CHEF TO EXPERIMENT IN THE KITCHEN.**

Once you've completed the cooking of the meat, you can then serve it taking into consideration the serving size. Bigger pieces have more calories and saturated fat. When cooking hamburger, 97% fat free means that 3% of what's there is fat, but this also means that 30% of the calories are fat calories. This was discussed in *How to Bypass Your Bypass*. Hamburger, which has more fat (eg. 80% lean, actually 20% of what's there is fat, and I don't even want to think about the number of fat calories) is even worse for you. Buy the leanest meat you can and cook it to let the grease run out of the meat and away from you. For those of you interested in meat substitutes there are a number of these which are great protein sources with less fat than hamburger. These include soy and sunflower mixes, Seitan, and textured vegetable protein (TVP) which can be added to marinara (tomato sauces) to provide a hamburger-like taste and texture. You might be surprised, but some pizzas have this added to them to add protein and reduce the amount of saturated fat.

Other considerations for main menu items include pasta dishes, rice, beans, et cetera. Most of these can be accomplished with little or no preparation time. The exception to this is the preparation of beans. All beans should be thoroughly examined to remove any which look damaged. Then they should be placed in a saucepan and covered with water for 8 to 12 hours, this will allow them time to absorb water before cooking them. You can do this in the morning and then go about your daily routine. Any beans that float when you first put them in the water should be removed and thrown away. Lentils and split peas do not need to be soaked. After 8 to 12 hours drain the beans and cover with enough water to bring the water level one inch above the beans. Bring to a simmer and skim off any foam/residue. Then boil for about 10 minutes. The beans are now ready for the recipe you will be using them in.

The next consideration is (are) the vegetable(s). One of the problems people have here is the same difficulty they have with the rest of their cooking; namely, limited experience with more than one approach to preparing something. Many people pour a can of vegetables into a pan, or from a bag, and boil the vegetables to death. Not only do the vegetables lose their color and appeal, but the nutrients (all those vitamins and minerals we buy pills to replace) go right down the drain with the water.

THE DIET MYTH

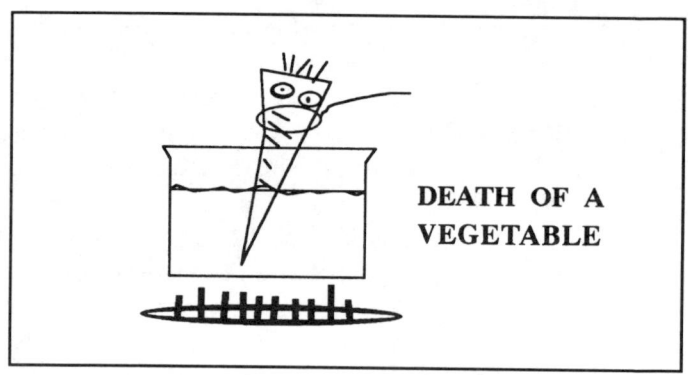

DEATH OF A VEGETABLE

Whenever possible use fresh vegetables, then frozen and then canned. Canned items should be drained and rinsed to remove as much of the salt and preservatives added to them as possible. You know, the salt, monosodium glutamate, and everything else you could possibly think of. Speaking of salt, there is a company called "MRS GRIMES" which cans beans. The entire can has only 560 milligrams (mgs) of sodium compared with 1575 mgs in many other (equal-sized cans) brands. This just goes to show, that just because it's canned, it doesn't have to be loaded with salt. Again, I don't own any stock in this company, my wife was the one who found it. I'm just letting you know.

Once you decide on vegetables, and I still consider potatoes a good vegetable, you need to decide how to prepare it. Some can be eaten raw, others steamed. You can even grill vegetables. Remember, before you eat fresh fruits and vegetables, wash them. Except for bananas, peal them. You want to remember to clean all the dirt and everything else out of what you're eating and of course do this with clean, uncontaminated water. I've been to some very expensive restaurants that had wonderful looking salads, only to bite into them and find out someone hadn't washed them. WASH YOUR FRUITS AND VEGETABLES THOROUGHLY BEFORE EATING THEM TO REMOVE THE DIRT AND BACTERIA, AND COOK YOUR MEAT. YOU DON'T HAVE TO TURN IT BLACK, BUT IF IT'S STILL BLEEDING, SOMETHING ELSE MIGHT BE ALIVE TOO – YOU KNOW, LIKE BACTERIA.

CLEAN AND COOK YOUR FOOD THOROUGHLY.

Fruits make an excellent contribution to menus while reducing calories and fats and providing a good source of carbohydrates. They help make great-tasting salads and side-dishes, and are good snack choices for us and our children. Remember, the idea really isn't to fill a number of boxes on a food pyramid, weight watchers plan or other scheme, but to get the right amount of calories, protein, carbohydrates and non-saturated fats in the food we eat. Each day doesn't have to be perfect and mistakes are made along the way. These shouldn't make you or anyone else feel like a failure. Desserts aren't necessarily no-nos, but they don't have to be a daily event either. When you eat them you have to consider the calories, fat, carbohydrates and (?) protein in them. If you find something with zero calories (besides water) let me know, the world's waiting to hear from you.

For other ideas and general recipe ideas I would again like to recommend my first book called *How to Bypass Your Bypass: What Your Doctor Doesn't Tell You About Cholesterol and Your Diet*. During the last five years I have been working with food producers and different restaurants in an effort to improve the quality of food available to you, while preserving the taste and appeal of the food. It was only a matter of time before this would lead to the development of new recipes for you and your family. The following chapter is dedicated to all of you who don't want to gain the average 7 to 10 pounds during the holidays, but don't want to feel like Scrooge either.

Chapter Eleven.
Healthy Happy Holiday Eating.

Eating with friends and family, or someone you've just met, has long been a way for people to socialize. This is never more true than during the Holiday Season when we catch up on what's happening with our closest friends and return home for the holidays to spend time with family members, many of whom we haven't seen for some time. Unfortunately, most people will gain 7 to 10 pounds from late November to early January and spend the rest of the year regretting it. For all too many people this time of year (along with other holidays) becomes one they wish wouldn't come. For other people who eat because "they like to" it is their family members who worry because of health concerns. In frustration many people will pick up one book after another, or order some diet plan they've seen on television, heard on radio or seen in the newspaper. These dietary gimmicks are designed to get your attention by promising quick weight loss, only to have the weight return later, leading to more guilt and frustration. Not so good for the dieter, but great for the diet industry and fad diets.

While we celebrate this time of year for different reasons, the additional food we eat can have some devastating effects on our weight and health. To do that we have divided this chapter into two sections. The first part will show what happens when you eat a typical holiday meal with all the creams, butter, et cetera. We will then make some subtle, yet important, changes and compare the differences. The latter part of this chapter was written to give you some healthy, yet appetizing ideas, so you can enjoy the Holiday Season without feeling like Scrooge in addition to the Healthier Holiday Meal you can use for those special events. The objective of this chapter is to give you ideas you can use to reduce the calories and saturated fat you're eating this year as well as illustrate certain principles to help you eat healthier all year long. By the way, even though these recipes taste great and are better for you, you still have to exercise (maybe that too) some self-control. Even I can't give you a recipe for a cheesecake which can be eaten by one person without paying for it calorie wise.

Unlike many individuals who try to convince you they are both master chefs as well as physician/nutritionist, et cetera, I am not a master chef. These recipes are provided by friends and family members who have searched their files to find tasty recipes which are good for you. As I continue to collect these recipes, I have continued to learn and I hope you will also. We hope you will enjoy several of these choices and share them with family and friends. Happy Holidays!!'

THE TYPICAL HOLIDAY MEAL/GATHERING

Turkey with Dressing (Stuffing)
Bread with Butter
Potatoes and Gravy
Cranberries
Green Bean Casserole
Sweet Potatoes
Peas with Butter
Egg Nog
Dessert: Pumpkin Pie and Pecan Pie

THE HEALTHIER HOLIDAY MEAL/GATHERING

Turkey (Roasted) without Dressing
Wild Rice Casserole in the Place of Turkey Stuffing
Honey Whole Grain Bread
Mashed Potatoes with Garlic
Cranberries
Steamed Green Beans
Steamed Carrots
Twice Baked Sweet Potatoes
Hot Cranberry Brew
Dessert: Orange Chantilly

For many people turkey is what we associate with the holidays. As a child growing up, I can still remember the smell of turkey cooking in the oven at my grandmother's house. You knew everything was almost ready when you could smell the turkey. For many years, people have been told that turkey was better for them than "red meat." However, many people didn't like the flavor of turkey and found it to be too dry, mostly because they tend to over cook it. Many companies began adding fat to their turkeys and other meats to lure people to eat turkey throughout the year. The important thing about selecting a turkey is to find one that is **unbasted**, ie. without the added fat. Turkey prepared properly will not be dried out and you don't need the added fat to make it taste good.

When roasting turkey, chicken, cornish game hens, duck, goose or anything else, you want to place the bird on a rack which then sits in a pan. This allows the oils/fats from the bird to drain away rather than having the bird sit in fat while it is in the oven. This is probably one of the simplest foods to prepare. After cleaning the bird thoroughly and removing the package with heart, kidneys, et cetera, you are ready to roast. The amount of time you need to cook a turkey is dependent upon the weight. As a general rule turkeys are roasted at 325 degrees Fahrenheit with aluminum foil placed over the top of the bird to prevent burning the top in conventional ovens. The foil should be removed for the last 45 minutes of roasting. The cooking time is less in a convection oven which cooks from top and bottom, hence, reducing the cooking time. Once the turkey is cooked and ready for carving, the skin should be removed to get rid of excess fat and calories.

Table 1. Estimated cooking time for turkey

Weight (Pounds)	Hours cooking time
6 to 8	3.5 to 4.0
8 to 12	4.0 to 4.5
12 to 16	4.5 to 5.5
16 to 20	5.5 to 6.5
20 to 24	6.5 to 7.5

When completely cooked the meat thermometer should read 185 degrees Fahrenheit. Some birds have pop-up thermometers which show when cooking is completed. Remember, it's better to be safe than sorry and meat should never be left out at room temperature unless you like visiting emergency rooms.

Meat servings, no matter what they are or how much you like them, should be about 3 ounces. This is roughly the size of a stack of playing cards. The following is the nutritional value of a serving of turkey.

THE COMPARISON

THE TYPICAL HOLIDAY MEAL/GATHERING

The Turkey
For this part of the recipes we will roast the turkey the same way – on a rack above the pan so the turkey is not sitting in the grease it is cooking in. The difference, however, will be in the type of turkey you choose to cook.

TRADITIONAL OVEN BAKED TURKEY

Recipe By: Diane M. Fleming
Serving Size: 3 ounces
Preparation Time: 6:00

Thoroughly clean the turkey with cold running tap water to remove debris and trim away excess fat. Remove the giblets (discard) and other packaged material from the cavity of the bird. The turkey should be placed in a rack which is then placed inside a roasting pan. The oven should be preheated to 325 degrees Fahrenheit. Once the oven is ready, place aluminum foil over the top of the turkey and bake. Remove the foil during the last 45 minutes of cooking. Cool for approximately 15 minutes before carving.

Per serving: 108 Calories; 5g Fat (47% calories from fat); 14g Protein (52% calories from protein); 0g Carbohydrate; 46mg Cholesterol; 44mg Sodium

TURKEY STUFFING

Recipe By: a Grandmother
Serving Size: 20

Ingredients
1	large	onion
1	large	celery stalk
2	medium	eggs
2	teaspoons	poultry seasoning
1	teaspoon	salt
1/4	teaspoon	pepper
16	cups	dry bread crumbs
4	cups	water
1	cup	raisins

Mix all the ingredients together in a food grinder until consistency is reached for stuffing mix. Refrigerate overnight. Once the turkey has been thoroughly cleaned and prepared for roasting, the cavity of the bird should be filled with the stuffing. This will be cooked with the turkey. The remainder of the stuffing should be baked in the oven at 350 degrees Fahrenheit for 3 hours. During this time the pan should be covered to keep moist.

Per serving: 122 Calories; 2g Fat (12% calories from fat); 3g (10% calories from Protein); 24g Carbohydrate (78% calories from carbohydrate); 0mg Cholesterol; 305mg Sodium.

BASIC WHITE BREAD

Serving Size: 16
Preparation Time: 3:00

Ingredients

1	package	active baker's yeast
1	teaspoon	sugar
1 1/4	cups	water – lukewarm
6	cups	all-purpose flour
2	tablespoons	sugar
2	teaspoons	salt
1	cup	milk
3	tablespoons	butter

Add one teaspoon sugar to 1/4 cup lukewarm water and stir to dissolve. Sprinkle yeast over water and let soften one minute. Stir into water and "proof" for 15 minutes. Mixture should rise slightly and become bubbly.

Heat remaining water with butter and milk until the butter melts. Cool this mixture to lukewarm. Mix three cups flour, 2 tbsp sugar, and salt in a large bowl. Beat in yeast mixture and buttermilk mixture. Gradually stir in enough of the remaining flour to form a soft dough, using 5-1/5 to 6-1/2 cups flour altogether.

Turn dough onto floured surface and allow to rest a minute. Knead until smooth and elastic, about 10 minutes. Place in a greased bowl, turning to grease all sides. Cover with a damp tea towel and allow to rise in a warm place until double in bulk, about one hour.

Punch down dough, kneading it until it is about its original size. Return to bowl, cover, and allow to rise again until double in bulk, about 1-1/2 hours. Turn out onto lightly floured surface. Divide dough in half and shape each half into a loaf to fit an 8-1/2" x 4-1/2" pan. Place in greased pans, cover, and allow to rise in a warm place for one hour.

Bake at 400 degrees for 25-30 minutes. When done, bread will be well browned and shrunken in from sides. Remove from pans and cool on wire racks.

Per serving: 208 Calories; 3g Fat (14% calories from fat); 6g Protein (12% calories from protein); 39g Carbohydrate (74% calories from carbohydrate); 8mg Cholesterol; 298mg Sodium

1 tablespoon (pat) butter per slice of bread

Per serving: 100 Calories; 11g Fat (100% calories from fat); 0g Protein; 0g Carbohydrate; 31mg Cholesterol; 116mg Sodium.

MASHED POTATOES

Serving Size: 4
Preparation Time: 1:00

Ingredients

4	whole	potatoes
1/2	cup	hot milk
2	tablespoons	butter – melted
1	teaspoon	salt
1/4	teaspoon	black pepper
2	whole	eggs

Boil potatoes until tender. Mash with 1/4 cup milk, butter, salt, and pepper. Beat in eggs and remaining milk. Beat eggs and milk into potatoes until fluffy. Serve at once.

Per serving: 167 Calories; 9g Fat (47% calories from fat); 5g Protein (12% calories from protein); 17g Carbohydrate (41% calories from carbohydrate); 110mg Cholesterol; 638mg Sodium.

TURKEY GRAVY

Serving Size: 12
Preparation Time: 0:45

Ingredients

1/2	pound	turkey giblets
1/2	cup	all-purpose flour
2	whole	eggs – chopped
1	package	turkey livers

Place turkey giblets into saucepan. Add enough water to cover and salt lightly. Cover and bring to a simmer for 1 hour or until tender. Add the turkey livers and simmer approximately 20 to 30 minutes until livers are tender. Remove the giblets and liver and chop up.

Add enough water to the reserved broth (still in the saucepan) to make 3 cups. In a separate container combine 1 cup of the broth mixture with the flour and pepper. Mix thoroughly. Now combine the flour mixture and remaining turkey broth. Cook and stir until thickened and bubbling. Continue cooking for an additional 1 to 2 minutes. Stir in the chopped giblets and liver. Finally, stir in the chopped up hard-boiled eggs. Heat thoroughly.

Per serving: 88 Calories; 3g Fat (27% calories from fat); 10g Protein (45% calories from protein); 5g Carbohydrate (28% calories from carbohydrate); 201mg Cholesterol; 50mg Sodium.

CRANBERRY SAUCE

Recipe By: Diane M. Fleming
Serving Size: 10
Preparation Time: 0:30

Ingredients

1	cup	sugar
1/2	cup	water
1/2	cup	orange juice
1	tablespoon	orange zest
3	cups	cranberries

Mix the water, sugar, orange juice and orange zest in a saucepan and stir to dissolve. Bring to a boil and add the cranberries. Return to a boil and then reduce heat to boil gently for about 10 minutes, stirring occasionally. Remove and cool to room temperature. Then refrigerate to chill before serving.

Per serving: 96 Calories; less than one gram Fat (1% calories from fat); 0g Protein; 25g Carbohydrate (99% calories from carbohydrate); 0mg Cholesterol; 1mg Sodium.

GREEN BEAN CASSEROLE

Serving Size: 6
Preparation Time: 0:40

Ingredients

10 3/4	ounces	cream of mushroom soup
3/4	cup	milk
1/8	teaspoon	pepper
18	ounces	green beans
2 3/4	ounces	french fried onions

Mix the soup, milk, pepper, green beans and 1/2 the can of french fried onions together in a casserole dish. Place in a preheated oven for 30 minutes at 350 degrees Fahrenheit. After 30 minutes remove from the oven and top with the remaining onions. Bake for an additional 5 minutes or until onions are golden brown.

Per serving: 77 Calories; 3.6g Fat (37% calories from fat); 3g Protein (16% calories from protein); 9.5g Carbohydrate (47% calories from carbohydrate); 5mg Cholesterol; 234mg Sodium.

SWEET POTATOES

Serving Size: 6
Preparation Time: 1:30

Ingredients

6	medium	sweet potatoes
1/4	cup	brown sugar – firmly packed
1/2	cup	butter
	pinch	nutmeg
1/2	teaspoon	grated orange peel
1	cup	apple – peeled and chopped

Preheat the oven to 375 degrees Fahrenheit. Puncture the skins of the sweet potatoes (yams) with a fork to allow steam to escape while cooking. Bake for 30 to 45 minutes, until tender to fork. Cut a thin slice (lengthwise) from the top of each sweet potato and scoop out the inside of each, leaving a thin shell behind. Set the shells to the side for later. Mix the sweet potatoes, brown sugar, butter, nutmeg and orange peel together. Mix at a medium speed until no lumps remain. Stir the apple pieces in by hand.

Place the potato shells onto a cooking sheet sprayed with no-stick cooking spray. Fill each shell with the mixture and bake for 15 to 20 minutes until thoroughly heated.

Per serving: 265 Calories; 15g Fat (51% calories from fat); 2g Protein (3% calories from protein); 31g Carbohydrate (46% calories from carbohydrate); 41mg Cholesterol; 169mg Sodium.

SWEET PEAS

Serving Size: 4
Preparation Time: 0:10

Ingredients

8	ounces	peas, frozen
2	tablespoons	butter

Bring 1/2 cup of water to a boil and add the frozen peas. Return to a boil, cover and simmer for 4 to 6 minutes until tender. Drain off water and mix in butter. Serve hot.

Per serving: 94 Calories; 6g Fat (55% calories from fat); 3g Protein (13% calories from protein); 8g Carbohydrate (32% calories from carbohydrate); 15mg Cholesterol; 121mg Sodium.

EGGNOG

Serving Size: 14
Preparation Time: 0:30

Ingredients

1	cup	rum
1	cup	cognac
1	pint	sweet cream
1	pint	whole milk
6	medium	eggs
1	cup	powdered sugar
	pinch	nutmeg

Separate the eggs. Set aside the egg yolks in a container in the refrigerator. In a large mixing bowl, beat the egg yolks, sugar, rum, cognac, milk, and cream until smooth. Chill in refrigerator overnight. When ready to serve, put the refrigerated rum mixture into a punch bowl. Beat the egg whites until stiff and fold them into the refrigerated rum mixture. Sprinkle nutmeg on top.

Per serving: 239 Calories; 12g Fat (62% calories from fat); 4g Protein (7% calories from protein); 12g Carbohydrate (31% calories from carbohydrate); 112mg Cholesterol; 53mg Sodium.

PUMPKIN PIE

Serving Size: 8
Preparation Time: 1:15

Ingredients

1/2	batch	pie pastry – enough for a 9" pie
2	cups	mashed pumpkin
2/3	cup	brown sugar
1	teaspoon	ground ginger
1/2	teaspoon	nutmeg
1	teaspoon	cinnamon
2	medium	eggs – beaten
3/4	cup	light cream

Roll out pastry and line a 9" pie pan with it. Bake at 450 degrees for 10 minutes. Cool shell. Combine pumpkin, sugar, and spices. Beat in eggs and cream. If desired, stir in rum. Bake at 325 degrees for 1 hour or until a knife inserted into pie comes clean.

Per serving: 186 Calories; 8g Fat (42% calories from fat); 3g Protein (6% calories from protein); 22g Carbohydrate (52% calories from carbohydrate); 66mg Cholesterol; 46mg Sodium

This is without topping or ice cream so don't forget to add these to the rest of the calories and fat.

PECAN PIE

Serving Size: 6
Preparation Time: 1:20

Ingredients

3	whole	eggs – beaten
1	cup	dark corn syrup
1	cup	sugar
1	teaspoon	vanilla extract
1/4	teaspoon	cinnamon
1	cup	pecans
1		9 inch pie crust – unbaked

Combine all ingredients and pour into unbaked pie shell. Bake at 325 degrees for one hour.

Per serving: 513 Calories; 17g Fat (28% calories from fat); 5g Protein (4% calories from protein); 91g Carbohydrate (68% calories from carbohydrate); 90mg Cholesterol; 306mg Sodium

This is without topping or ice cream so don't forget to add these to the rest of the calories and fat.

Well while this probably has your mouth watering right now, lets see how much **one serving** of each of these adds up to.

THE DIET MYTH

Table 2. The total cost of the Typical Holiday Meal.

Dish	Calories	Fat Grams	Protein Grams	Carbohydrate Grams
Turkey	108	5	14	0
Stuffing	122	2	3	24
Bread	208	3	6	39
Butter	100	1	0	0
Potatoes	167	9	5	17
Gravy	88	3	10	5
Cranberries	96	0	0	25
Green Bean Casserole	77	3.6	3	9.5
Sweet Potatoes	265	15	2	31
Sweet Peas	94	6	3	8
Eggnog	239	12	4	12
Pumpkin Pie	186	8	3	22
Pecan Pie	513	17	5	91
Total	**2263**	**94.6 (38%)**	**58 (10%)**	**283.5(52%)**

In total, this one holiday meal (again this is only one serving and doesn't include the nibbling and second courses everyone is so fond of) included a total of 2,263 calories including almost 95 grams of fat, 58 grams of protein and 283 grams of carbohydrates. It's easy to see why we gain 7 to 10 pounds each holiday. Now let's see if we can still have the types of foods we like without paying for it with our health/life.

TRADITIONAL OVEN BAKED TURKEY

Recipe By: Diane M. Fleming
Serving Size: 3 ounces
Preparation Time: 6:00
Categories: Main Entree

Thoroughly clean the turkey with cold running tap water to remove debris and trim away excess fat. Remove the giblets (discard) and other packaged material from the cavity of the bird. The turkey should be placed in a rack which is then placed inside a roasting pan. The oven should be preheated to 325 degrees Fahrenheit. Once the oven is ready, place aluminum foil over the top of the turkey and bake. Remove the foil during the last 45 minutes of cooking. Cool for approximately 15 minutes before carving.

Per serving: 108 Calories; 5g Fat (47% calories from fat); 14g Protein (52% calories from protein); 0g Carbohydrate; 46mg Cholesterol; 44mg Sodium.

WILD RICE CASSEROLE

Recipe By: Diane M. Fleming
Serving Size: 6
Preparation Time: 2:30

Ingredients

2	cups	wild rice – rinsed
1 1/2	teaspoons	salt
1/4	cup	corn oil
1	large	onion – coarsely chopped
6	medium	scallions – thinly sliced
3	large	celery stalks – coarsely chopped
2	medium	carrots – coarsely chopped
1	teaspoon	marjoram – crumbled
1/2	teaspoon	rosemary – crumbled
1/2	teaspoon	thyme – crumbled
1/2	teaspoon	pepper – freshly ground
1	pound	fresh mushrooms – thinly sliced
2	tablespoons	unsalted butter
3	tablespoons	all-purpose flour
1 2/3	cups	chicken stock
2	cups	melba toast cubes
7	cups	water

In a large saucepan combine the rice, salt and water. Bring mixture to a boil, then simmer until the rice is chewy (about 55 minutes). Drain the water off. In a skillet, heat the oil and add onions and celery and cook for 10 minutes. Then add the carrots and seasonings. Cover the skillet and cook for another 10 minutes. Remove the vegetables.

Preheat the oven to 350 degrees Fahrenheit. Add mushrooms to the skillet and cook for 7 minutes. Then add the mushrooms to the vegetables. Take your casserole pan and spray it with a no-stick cooking spray. Mix the flour and butter and combine with vegetable and rice mixture and the melba toast cubes. Place in casserole pan and bake for 1 hour.

Note: Excellent in the place of turkey stuffing. Serve this as a side dish.

Per serving: 374 Calories; 15g Fat (34% calories from fat); 12g Protein (13% calories from protein); 52g Carbohydrate (53% calories from carbohydrate); 11mg Cholesterol; 882mg Sodium.

HONEY WHOLE GRAIN BREAD

Recipe By: Diane M. Fleming
Serving Size: 20

Ingredients
3	cups	white flour
2	packages	dry yeast
1 1/2	teaspoons	salt
1	cup	water
1	cup	cottage cheese
4	tablespoons	butter
1/2	cup	honey
2		egg beaters® 99% egg substitute
2 1/2	cups	whole wheat flour
1/2	cup	rolled oats

In a saucepan heat the water, cottage cheese, butter and honey until warm (120-130 degrees Fahrenheit), then add yeast and the egg substitute and mix well. Add the wheat flour and rolled oats. Then stir in the white flour.

Kneed until smooth and elastic. Let rise until doubled. Punch down and shape loaves into bread pans which have been sprayed with no-stick cooking spray. Let rise for about 1 hour. Place in a preheated oven (350 degrees Fahrenheit) and bake for 35 to 40 minutes. Serve.

Per serving: 191 Calories; 3g Fat (14% calories from fat); 7g Protein (15% calories from protein); 35g Carbohydrate (71% calories from carbohydrate); 7mg Cholesterol; 248mg Sodium.

MASHED POTATOES WITH GARLIC

Recipe By: Diane M. Fleming
Serving Size: 4
Preparation Time: 1:00

Ingredients

4	whole	potatoes
1/2	cup	skim milk – hot
2	tablespoons	butter – melted
1	teaspoon	salt
1/4	teaspoon	black pepper
1	clove	garlic – roasted

Boil potatoes until tender. Mash with 1/4 cup milk, butter, salt, and pepper. Beat in eggs and remaining milk. Beat eggs and milk into potatoes until fluffy. Serve at once.

Per serving: 129 Calories; 6g Fat (40% calories from fat); 3g Protein (9% calories from protein); 17g Carbohydrate (51% calories from carbohydrate); 16mg Cholesterol; 612mg Sodium.

CRANBERRY SAUCE

Recipe By: Diane M. Fleming
Serving Size: 10
Preparation Time: 0:30

Ingredients

1	cup	sugar
1/2	cup	water
1/2	cup	orange juice
1	tablespoon	orange zest
3	cups	cranberries

Mix the water, sugar, orange juice and orange zest in a saucepan and stir to dissolve. Bring to a boil and add the cranberries. Return to a boil and then reduce heat to boil gently for about 10 minutes, stirring occasionally. Remove and cool to room temperature. Then refrigerate to chill before serving.

Per serving: 96 Calories; less than one gram Fat (1% calories from fat); 0g Protein; 25g Carbohydrate (99% calories from carbohydrate); 0mg Cholesterol; 1mg Sodium.

STEAMED GREEN BEANS

Serving Size: 4
Preparation Time: 0:10

Ingredients
16   ounces   green beans, frozen

Bring 1/2 cup of water to a boil and add the frozen green beans. Return to a boil, cover and simmer for 4 to 6 minutes until tender. Drain off water and serve hot.

Per serving: 15 Calories; 0g Fat; 1g Protein (27% calories from protein); 3g Carbohydrate (73% calories from carbohydrate); 0mg Cholesterol; 3mg Sodium.

STEAMED CARROTS

Serving Size: 4
Preparation Time: 0:10

Ingredients
16   ounces   carrots, frozen

Bring 1/2 cup of water to a boil and add the frozen carrots. Return to a boil, cover and simmer for 4 to 6 minutes until tender. Drain off water and serve hot.

Per serving: 21 Calories; 0g Fat; 0g Protein; 5g Carbohydrate (100% calories from carbohydrate); 0mg Cholesterol; 17mg Sodium.

TWICE-BAKED SWEET POTATOES

Recipe By: Alice Driscoll
Serving Size: 4
Preparation Time: 1:30

Ingredients

2	large	sweet potatoes
1/3	cup	egg substitute
1/2	cup	crushed pineapple in juice – drained (save juice)
1/2	cup	skim milk
1/3	cup	apple – finely chopped
	dash	paprika
	dash	parsley

Preheat the oven to 400 degrees Fahrenheit and spray the baking pan with no-stick cooking spray. Clean the sweet potatoes and cut (lenghwise) a groove along the top and puncture with a fork to allow steam to escape during cooking. Bake in the oven for approximately 45 to 50 minutes until tender to fork. Remove and cut in half lengthwise. Remove the sweet potato flesh and mix this with the egg substitute in a mixing bowl. Stir in the pineapple juice and skim milk (add slowly) until you reach stuffing consistency. Then stir in the pineapple and apple pieces. Stuff the sweet potato shells with the stuffing mixture. Sprinkle with paprika.

Bake for about 15 minutes and remove from oven. Sprinkle with parsley and serve.

Per serving: 116 Calories; 2g Fat (19% calories from fat); 4g Protein; 20g Carbohydrate; 1mg Cholesterol; 62mg Sodium.

HOT CRANBERRY BREW

Recipe By: Ellen Peterson
Serving Size: 8 ounces

Ingredients
1	cup	brown sugar
1 1/2	teaspoons	whole cloves
4		cinnamon sticks
2	quarts	cranberry juice
46	ounces	pineapple juice
4 1/2	cans	water

Mix ingredients together until hot. Serve.

Per serving: 161 Calories; less than one gram Fat (0% calories from fat); 0g Protein (2% calories from protein); 41g Carbohydrate (100% calories from carbohydrate); 0mg Cholesterol; 10mg Sodium.

ORANGE CHANTILLY

Recipe By: Richard M. Fleming
Serving Size: 12

Ingredients

1	cup	plain nonfat yogurt
1	cup	orange juice
1	cup	nonfat dairy whipped topping
1	box	sugar free orange gelatin

Drain the yogurt by placing it in cheese cloth and allowing it to drain for one hour. Prepare the gelatin according to package instructions and chill until set. Then whip with an electric mixer until it doubles in volume. It should have the consistency of whipped cream. Place the orange juice in a pan and bring to a boil. Then reduce the heat and simmer for about 20 minutes until a thick syrup remains – approximately 2 tablespoons worth. Mix the drained yogurt and orange syrup together, then gently add the jello mixture and whipped topping with a rubber spatula.

Per serving: 20 Calories; less than one gram Fat (0% calories from fat); 1g Protein (20% of calories from protein); 4g Carbohydrate (80% calories from carbohydrate); 0mg Cholesterol; 15mg Sodium.

Like the first Holiday meal, this too should leave you more than full and ready to compliment the chief. Lets take a look at the difference is nutritional values.

Table 3. A healthier approach to Holiday cooking.

Dish	Calories	Fat Grams	Protein Grams	Carbohydrate Grams
Turkey	108	5	14	0
Wild Rice Casserole	374	15	12	52
Bread	191	3	7	35
Mashed Potatoes	129	6	3	17
Cranberries	96	0	0	25
Green Beans	15	0	1	3
Carrots	21	0	0	5
Sweet Potatoes	116	2	4	20
Cranberry Drink	161	0	0	41
Orange Chantilly	20	0	1	4
Total	**1231**	**31 (23%)**	**42 (14%)**	**202 (66%)**

With each meal there was turkey, stuffing or rice substitute, bread, potatoes, cranberries, vegetables, sweet potatoes, a drink (non-alcoholic) and dessert. The difference doesn't lie in the taste or flavor of the food, but the nutritional value of the food. By changing the way in which we prepare the food we have cut the number of calories in half, reduced the fat to one-third of what we started out with, only reduced the amount of protein by one-quarter and cut more than 80 grams (325 calories) of carbohydrate from the meal. This is the type of food that can leave you satisfied both physically and mentally.

Lets look at one more comparison for our Jewish friends who will be celebrating Hanukkah and Rosh Hashana during the holiday season.

BRISKET

Recipe By: Evelyne Beninson
Serving Size: 16
Preparation Time: 3:00

Ingredients

3	pounds	brisket – flat cut
1	envelope	onion soup mix
3	cloves	garlic – minced
8	ounces	dry red wine
		pepper – to taste

Thoroughly clean the brisket and place it in a bowl which has a lid. Mix all four ingredients together (this is the marinade) and pour over the brisket. Marinade the brisket overnight, mixing the ingredients three to four times. If you do not have a mixing bowl with lid large enough to hold the brisket and marinade, a large zip lock bag can be used. You should check with your butcher or meat department where you shop, but the leaner briskets come from the loin region and will have fewer calories with less saturated fat, but taste just as good – maybe better.

Per serving: 284 Calories; 23g Fat (76% calories from fat); 15g Protein (21% calories from protein); 2g Carbohydrate (3% calories from carbohydrate); 62mg Cholesterol; 274mg Sodium.

This same recipe can be improved simply by selecting a leaner piece of meat.

BRISKET FROM SIRLOIN STEAK

Recipe By: Evelyne Beninson
Serving Size: 16
Preparation Time: 3:00

Ingredients

3	pounds	sirloin steak – flat cut
1	envelope	onion soup mix
3	cloves	garlic – minced
8	ounces	dry red wine
		pepper – to taste

The same recipe using sirloin steak instead of brisket cuts 90 calories and 11 grams of fat from each serving.

Per serving: 194 Calories; 12g Fat (61% calories from fat); 16g Protein (33% calories from protein); 2g Carbohydrate (6% calories from carbohydrate); 54mg Cholesterol; 262mg Sodium.

HEALTHIER (BUT NOT PERFECT) HOLIDAY (OR ANYTIME) RECIPES – IMPROVING ON OLDER RECIPES

APPLE CIDER STEW

Recipe By: Diane M. Fleming
Serving Size: 6
Preparation Time: 2:00

Ingredients

3	tablespoons	flour
2	teaspoons	salt
1/4	teaspoon	pepper
1/4	teaspoon	thyme
1	pound	beef stew meat
2	cups	apple cider
1/2	cup	water
2	tablespoons	vinegar
4	medium	carrot – quartered
3	medium	potato – peeled and diced
2	medium	onion – diced
1	stalk	celery – 1 inch pieces
1	medium	apple – cored and diced
1/2	cup	barley
1/4	cup	green beans

Combine the flour, salt, pepper and thyme in a paper bag. Add the meat and shake to coat. Pour 1/4 cup apple cider into Dutch oven and add beef. Heat until meat is browned. Add remaining cider, water and vinegar. Bring to a boil, then reduce heat and simmer for 1-1/2 to 2 hours, or until the meat is tender. Add the remainder of the ingredients and cook for 30 minutes or until the vegetables are tender.

Per serving: 417 Calories; 16g Fat (35% calories from fat); 25g Protein (24% calories from protein); 42g Carbohydrate (41% calories from carbohydrate); 76mg Cholesterol; 1145mg Sodium.

CABBAGE BURGERS

Recipe By: Jan Weeks
Serving Size: 20
Preparation Time: 0:00

Ingredients

2	cups	water – lukewarm
2		yeast cakes
2	teaspoons	salt
1/4	cup	sugar
4	cups	flour
1/4	cup	shortening
6	cups	cabbage – chopped fine
1	pound	ground beef
1/4	cup	onion – chopped fine

Dissolve the yeast in lukewarm water. Add the sugar, salt and shortening together along with 2 cups of flour. Beat well. Knead and gradually add the remaining 2 cups of flour. Place in oiled bowl and set in a warm place to rise for about one hour. Once the dough has doubled in size, knead and allow to double a second time.

Break up and brown the ground beef. Once browned, add cabbage and cook slowly until the cabbage is tender. Drain off excess grease and set aside to chill.

Once the bread dough has risen a second time it is time to fill the biscuits. Divide the dough in half, working with only half the dough at a time. Roll out the dough to a thickness of 1/4 to 1/2 inch. Cut dough into 5 inch squares. Place 1/3 cup of cabbage-meat filling in the center of each square. Bring together the corners of the dough and pinch closed at center. Place on a cookie sheet which has been sprayed with no-stick cooking spray. Place each square with the pinched side down. Allow to rise about 25 minutes in a warm place.

Preheat the oven to 375 degrees Fahrenheit. Bake for 25-30 minutes. Remove and serve hot.

Note: The fat can be reduced considerably by buying ground beef which is 95% fat free or better.

Per serving: 198 Calories; 9g Fat (41% calories from fat); 7g Protein (14% calories from protein); 23g Carbohydrate (45% calories from carbohydrate); 19mg Cholesterol; 240mg Sodium.

HEALTHY CORN CHOWDER

Recipe By: Evelyne Beninson
Serving Size: 10
Preparation Time: 1:00

Ingredients

4	cups	corn – fresh or frozen
1/2	tablespoon	butter
2	cups	onion – peeled and chopped
1	cup	celery – diced
4	ounces	ham slices, extra lean – diced
2	cloves	garlic – peeled and minced
21	ounces	chicken broth, low-sodium
2	cups	potatoes – raw, peeled, diced
1/4	cup	all-purpose flour
1/2	teaspoon	black pepper
1/8	teaspoon	ground red pepper
2	cups	skim milk
1	teaspoon	Worcestershire sauce

Mix 2 and 1/2 cups of the corn in a blender or food processor until smooth and then set aside. Melt the margarine in a Dutch oven using medium heat. Add the onions, celery, ham, garlic and sauté until the vegetables are tender (about 10 minutes), stirring occasionally. Then add the chicken broth and potatoes and bring to a boil. Reduce the heat to a simmer and cook for 20 minutes, stirring frequently. Add the 1 and 1/2 cups of corn and the pureed corn and cook for another 10 minutes.

In a separate bowl mix the flour and pepper together. Then slowly add the milk and Worcestershire sauce, blending with a wire wisk. Gradually add this mixture to the chowder in the Dutch oven. Continue cooking for another 10 minutes, stirring constantly until thickened.

Per serving: 138 Calories; 3g Fat (16% calories from fat); 9g Protein (26% calories from protein); 21g Carbohydrate (42% calories from carbohydrate); 8mg Cholesterol; 709mg Sodium.

HUMMUS SANDWICH

Recipe By: Richard M. Fleming
Serving Size: 1
Preparation Time: 0:05

Ingredients

1		pita pocket
1/4	cup	hummus
1	leaf	spinach
1	slice	tomato
1/4	cup	alfalfa sprouts
1	slice	zucchini
1	slice	green pepper
1	slice	red pepper
1	slice	onion
1	slice	cucumber

Cut top 1/4 from pita pocket and reserve for another use.* Open pocket and spread one side with hummus. Add remaining ingredients.

* Broiled pieces of pita bread are excellent for dipping extra hummus.

Per serving: 425 Calories; 7g Fat (15% calories from fat); 17g Protein (16% calories from protein); 79g Carbohydrate (69% calories from carbohydrate); 0mg Cholesterol; 1075mg Sodium.

APPETIZERS AND DESSERTS

APPLE CAKE

Recipe By:	Evelyne Beninson
Serving Size:	16
Preparation Time:	1:00

Ingredients

1/4	cup	butter
1	cup	sugar
1	medium	egg substitute
1	cup	all-purpose flour
1/2	cup	walnuts – coarsely chopped
1	teaspoon	cinnamon
1	teaspoon	nutmeg – freshly grated
1	teaspoon	baking soda
1/4	teaspoon	salt
3	medium	apples (grated) – cooked and peeled

Preheat the oven to 350 degrees Fahrenheit. Spray 8 inch square baking dish with no-stick cooking spray. Thoroughly mix the butter and sugar in a large mixing bowl. Beat in the egg substitute, then add the flour, walnuts, cinnamon, nutmeg, baking soda and salt. Mix thoroughly. Stir in the grated apples. Spoon the mixture into the prepared baking dish and bake for approximately 35 to 40 minutes until golden brown and toothpick inserted into the center comes out clean. Cool and cut into squares for serving.

Per serving: 133 Calories; 5g Fat (35% calories from fat); 3g Protein; 19g Carbohydrate; 8mg Cholesterol; 171mg Sodium.

APPLE LOKSHEN KUGEL (SWEET)

Recipe By: Evelyne Beninson
Serving Size: 20
Preparation Time: 1:30

Ingredients

8	ounces	egg noodles medium
1/8	cup	margarine – melted
4	egg	egg beaters® 99% egg substitute
3	medium	apples – chopped and peeled
1/4	cup	sugar
1 1/2	teaspoons	salt
2	teaspoons	cinnamon
1/2	teaspoon	vanilla

Cook and drain the noodles according to package directions. Place noodles in a large bowl and stir in margarine and egg beaters. Add the prepared apples and add along with the remainder of the ingredients. Mix well.

Preheat the oven to 350 degrees Fahrenheit. Pour the kugel mixture into a 9 by 13 inch pan which has been coated with no-stick cooking spray. Bake for 40 minutes to an hour, or until lightly browned.

Per serving: 42 Calories; 1g Fat (25% calories from fat); 1g Protein (10% calories from protein); 7g Carbohydrate (65% calories from carbohydrate); 0mg Cholesterol; 207mg Sodium.

BANANA BREAD (LOW-FAT)

Recipe By: Evelyne Beninson
Serving Size: 20
Preparation Time: 1:30

Ingredients

2	egg equivalent	Egg Beaters® 99% egg substitute
3/4	cup	sugar
1	cup	bananas – mashed
1/3	cup	buttermilk (could use kefir or yogurt)
1	tablespoon	vegetable oil
1	tablespoon	vanilla
1 3/4	cups	flour
2	teaspoons	baking powder
1/2	teaspoon	baking soda
1/2	teaspoon	salt

Preheat the oven to 325 degrees Fahrenheit and spray an 8.5 by 4.5 by 2.5 inch loaf pan with no stick cooking spray. Using an electric mixer, mix the egg substitute and sugar until thick but light. This should take about 5 minutes. Mix in the mashed (3) bananas, buttermilk, oil and vanilla. Sift the dry ingredients over the mixture and beat until blended. Pour into the pan and bake in the oven for 1 hour until the top is golden brown and toothpick comes out clean when placed into the center of the bread. Take out of oven and tip out onto cooling rack.

Per serving: 87 Calories; 1g Fat (8% calories from fat); 2g Protein (10% calories from protein); 18g Carbohydrate (82% calories from carbohydrate); 0mg Cholesterol; 138mg Sodium.

DIANE'S HOLIDAY CHEESECAKE
(To die for – not because of!)

Recipe By: Diane M. Fleming
Serving Size: 12
Preparation Time: 2:00 plus chill time
Categories: Dessert

Ingredients

3/4	cup	graham cracker crumbs – crushed
2	tablespoons	margarine – melted, reduced cal.
15	ounces	part-skim ricotta cheese
8	ounces	yogurt, skim milk non-fat
1	cup	sugar
2	tablespoons	all-purpose flour
2	tablespoons	lemon juice
8	ounces	light cream cheese – softened
6	ounces	egg substitute
2 1/2	teaspoons	vanilla
		Fresh fruit (strawberries, raspberries)

Combine the crushed graham crackers and margarine; press onto bottom of a 9-inch springform (cheesecake) pan. Bake for 5 minutes in a oven preheated to 325 degrees Fahrenheit. Cool.

In a blender combine the ricotta cheese, yogurt, sugar, flour and lemon juice. Cover and blend the mixture until smooth. Set aside. In a large mixing bowl beat or mix the cream cheese until smooth. Add the egg substitute and vanilla and beat on low speed until combined, then mix on high speed until smooth. Slowly add ricotta cheese mixture to cream cheese mixture, mixing on low speed until combined. Pour onto crust.

Place on a shallow baking pan in an oven preheated to 325 degrees. Bake for one hour or until the center is nearly set when shaken gently. Cool for 15 minutes. Loosen the crust from the sides of the pan. Cool for another 30 minutes and remove the sides of the pan. Cool completely and chill for 4 to 6 hours. Top with fresh fruit.

Per serving: 236 Calories; 10g Fat (39% calories from fat); 9g Protein (15% calories from protein); 27g Carbohydrate (46% calories from carbohydrate); 22mg Cholesterol; 197mg Sodium.

LEMON YOGURT COOKIES

Recipe By: Richard M. Fleming
Serving Size: 30

Ingredients

1 1/4	cups	all-purpose flour
1/2	teaspoon	baking soda
1/2	cup	lemon yogurt, lowfat
1/2	cup	almonds – toasted and chopped
1/2	cup	granulated sugar
1/4	cup	packed brown sugar
1	egg	Egg Beaters® 99% egg substitute
1	teaspoon	vanilla

Spray a cookie sheet with no-stick cooking spray. Preheat the oven to 375 degrees Fahrenheit. Beat yogurt, vanilla and egg substitute together, then add the flour, baking soda, almonds and sugars. Beat well. Drop onto the cookie sheet 2 inches apart and place into the oven for 8 to 10 minutes until done. Remove and cool.

Per serving: 49 Calories; 1g Fat (11% calories from fat); 1g Protein (8% calories from protein); 10g Carbohydrate (81% calories from carbohydrate); 0mg Cholesterol; 30mg Sodium.

In the end, our recipes are like our lives: we get out of them what we put into them. Like the old Chinese proverb that says: *If we don't change the direction we're going, we will end up where we're headed.* Hopefully, these recipes, like the book, has caused you to think about the way you eat and what you put into your body. If it has done so, then it has succeeded.

Chapter Twelve.
If We Don't Change the Direction We're Going, We Will End Up Where We're Headed.

Centuries ago a Chinese philosopher summed it up pretty nicely when he said, "If We Don't Change the Direction We're Going, We Will End Up Where We're Headed." Today the number one cause of death in THE WORLD is heart disease not infection, war, famine, cancer or anything else. Thousands of years ago people lived long lives without the aid of modern medicine or modern food. Muhammad lived for 62 years (570-632 AD), Gandhi lived for 79 years (1869-1948 AD), Buddha for 80 years (563-483 BC) and Methuselah for 969 years. Regardless of race, creed, color, or religion, people have been able to live long, healthy, productive lives as long as they took good care of themselves. Those who didn't take good care of themselves died young.

Many people today assume that they can eat whatever they want, smoke whatever they want, drink whatever they want and sit around as much as they want. When they have a problem they simply go to their doctor (or someone else) and they will get a magic pill which will take the problem away. This way of thinking has resulted in charlatans selling all sorts of promises and potions to cure all the ills the medical doctors can't treat. In the Wild West, Medicine Shows traveled the country selling potions which had no benefit except for the profit it brought the peddler. Today with newsprint, television, radio and even the internet, these charlatans can sell products to you with claims that have no scientific proof, but all the charm and salability of a circus. W.C. Fields once said, "there's a sucker born every minute," and these diet gimmicks look at everyone that way.

The unfortunate problem is that people are so desperate to find a quick and easy solution to their health and medical problems that they have opened themselves up to these "con artists" who have no legal responsibilities because they don't guarantee success and because they're not medical doctors. Even some medical doctors have proclaimed they have the magic cure by telling you that if you only will become a vegetarian your heart and cholesterol problems will go away. While there is some initial benefit, the long-term (more than 18 months) results aren't as promising, but you don't hear about these results.

To make the point blatantly obvious, there are other doctors who will tell you that eating only meat is the answer. The problem is that there is no scientific proof to support the long-term use of these extremist diets, diet supplements or other gimmicks. The manufacturers of diet gimmicks, including vitamin supplements, powders and drinks, know they're not regulated by the Food and Drug Administration. So by law, they are not required to prove the safety or benefit of their product. One of the reasons the FDA came into existence was to crack down on some of the more obvious problems. For example, before the FDA there was a pill that you could take that "guaranteed" that you would lose weight, and IT DID. The problem was that once you stopped taking the pill you still continued to lose weight. What a great pill you say! Maybe, until you discover that people started dying from malnutrition. The FDA was finally able to get involved because of the problems. What did they discover? Inside the pill were "eggs" – not just any eggs, but the eggs of tapeworms. The tapeworms ate the food and the person starved to death. The tapeworms would grow so long that they would come out of the person. Not a pleasant thought, but indicative of the risks we take when there is no control over what we're sold by these people who would make a profit from our health problems without being held accountable.

WHY THE PROBLEM?

What's happened in the United States, Western Europe and now the rest of the world is no surprise if we look at what has happened during the last century. Before 1928 and the discovery of penicillin (antibiotic) by Sir Alexander Fleming, the greatest threat to survival was infectious disease. Food was scarce and people worked hard, using up most of the calories they ate in a day. Only the very wealthy had more than enough food to eat, and this lead to many of these people becoming obese. Food could not be preserved for long periods of time and there was little extra in the home to munch on all day long.

By 1940, penicillin becomes available and the death rate of soldiers from infections dramatically decreases during World War II. During and following the 1940s, technology changed dramatically and machines did much of the work that people used to do. Leisure time and prosperity leads to many people having an abundance of food and time to relax. We learn to preserve food by hydrogenation which results in more fats and calories in the food we eat. It is this fat (saturated) and calories which will cause our cholesterol levels to increase, as well as our risk of stroke, diabetes, risk of certain cancers and weight problems. Failure to recognize this will result in more and more health problems until medications are developed to try to treat these problems. Some of the medications (phen-fen), while designed to help, will be shown to create more problems. Other medications designed to lower cholesterol, have helped but are limited in what they can do because people refuse to make the changes in what they eat – expecting the medications to correct their problem. It was not until we presented our research in England (in the Fleming conference room of the Queen Elizabeth II Conference Center), in 1995, that the benefit of changing the diet with or without these medicines was known, and the importance of limiting the calories and saturated fat was proven scientifically.

Many of the health problems we face today are caused by ourselves and not some problem with the genes our parents gave us. After all, these same genes didn't kill our ancestors so why should they be killing us. Immigrants to this country die from heart disease and strokes that never affected their parents. The answer is quite simple! We're doing something different than our parents and grandparents did. In fact, we're doing a number of things differently. First of all, we're less active, so we need fewer calories than they did. Too many calories (regardless of whether they start out as protein, carbohydrates or fat) get stored in the body as extra fat. This can eventually lead to certain types of cancer, diabetes and along with the extra salt in our diet, high blood pressure. This extra fat gets stored as triglycerides and turned into cholesterol, which plugs up the arteries of our heart, brain and elsewhere until we have heart attacks, strokes or lose toes, feet, and even legs, particularly in your diabetic. This is easier today because along with our poor diets and lack of exercise, we smoke. This causes our blood vessels to spasm and blood clots to form, thereby reducing – if not totally blocking – blood flow from getting where it needs to go.

Secondly, the amount of "saturated fat" drives the production of cholesterol in our bodies. After all, if you give your body a lot of something and tell it to store it in the only way it can, your body will do just that, and the continued build up of cholesterol in the arteries of your body results in poorer blood flow where it wasn't too good to begin with. This is happening at younger and younger ages. As of 1995, 14.5 million girls and 13.1 million boys (25.6 million children) under age 19 had elevated cholesterol levels. This increase has been ignored for more than 30 years while we continue to bury our head in the sand, and prepare to bury our children at the same time. Poor dietary practices (junk food) and limited exercise has placed our children at greater risk for strokes, heart attacks, diabetes, obesity, cancer and high blood pressure problems than we are. Today 25 to 35% of our children have high cholesterol, high blood pressure, diabetes or are overweight.

This increase in cholesterol build up causes damage to the arteries of the body as shown in the following figure. This theory (The Fleming Unified Theory of Vascular Disease) shows how the build up of cholesterol on the arteries of the body from excess calories and/or saturated fat leads to narrowing (damage) of arteries throughout the body and not just the arteries of the heart. In some people this can be worsened by high homocysteine, fibrinogen or lipoprotein (a) levels which can increase the build up of cholesterol or increase the tendency to develop a blood clot in these damaged arteries. Within the arteries, the body will try to deal with the damage and when enough cholesterol has built up over time, the artery will become sufficiently damaged (inflammation) and bacterial (possibly other infection as well) can enter and grow causing further damage. These inflections may then lead to further damage. If we use antibiotics inappropriately (for viruses) or if the bacteria become resistant to the antibiotics we use, the next wave of infections to kill us may come from our cholesterol build up in the arteries of our neck and heart.

Many people are unaware of the effect this is having on children, women and minorities. This is not just a problem for white men over 50. As of 1995, there were more women who died from heart disease than anything else. In fact, more women (550,440) died from heart disease than men (455,152). During the same year 43,844 women died from breast cancer, while more than twice as many (96,428) died from strokes. While 1 in 8 or 9 women develop breast cancer, 1 in 5 women will have a heart attack or stroke. While similar dietary factors appear to play a role for many people, we continue to ignore the warnings and change what we eat and how we're living. Once a woman has a heart attack, 44% will die within one year, while 27% of the men will die in that same year.

Figure 1. Fleming Unified Theory of Vascular Disease.

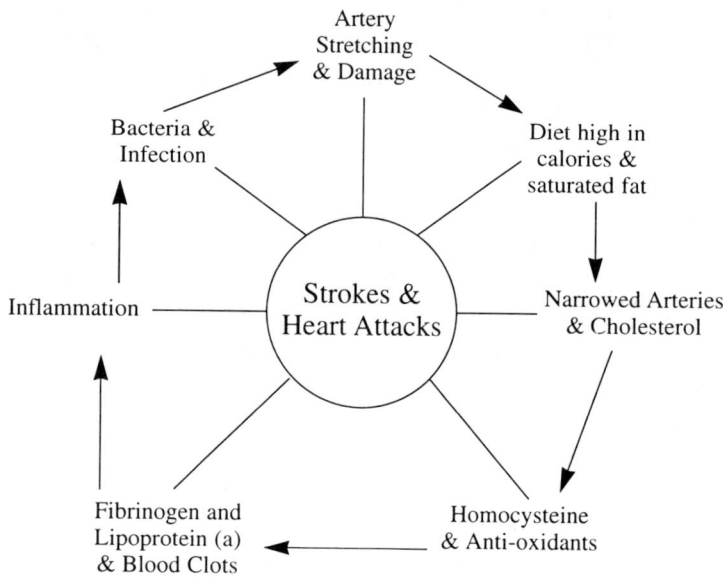

The problems appear to be greater for African-American women who have a 35.3% higher death rate from heart disease and 71.4% higher death rate from stroke, than white women. When we adjust for age, black women have a 71% higher death rate from heart disease than white women between the age of 35 and 74.

The average cholesterol level for women from 35-44 years of age is 195 mg/dl. Total cholesterol levels greater than 200 is accepted by most as too high. Yet research that has been published clearly agrees that cholesterol greater than 150 places a person at increased risk for strokes and heart attacks. As of 1995, there were almost 51 million women in the United States over age 20 who had cholesterol levels over 200. Of these, 53% of the non-Hispanic white women, 46% of the non-Hispanic black women, and 43% of the Mexican-American women had cholesterol levels higher than 200.

WE'RE IN A RAT RACE AND THE RATS ARE WINNING

Today the pace of our society has changed much of the way in which we approach everything. Unfortunately, for many people it has become an excuse to justify poor eating and exercise habits. We've gotten too used to blaming other people for our problems and not exercising self-control or planning far enough in advance to take care of problems before they occur.

There is no magic bullet which will take care of all of our health-care problems, no magic mineral or vitamin, powder or supplement. In many ways this is good, because it means that balancing what you eat and what you do is more important than depending upon someone's gimmick that will result in their making money off your problem.

Learning how much your body needs in a day is the first important step. As we've discussed, most people need 10 calories per pound per day, so if you want to weigh 140 pounds, you need to eat no more than 1400 calories in a day. If you eat 2000 calories a day, you won't weigh 140 lbs. I know and you know you're not going to sit down and figure out the amount of calories you eat in everything, but you need to have a good idea, otherwise you're going to continue doing what you're doing now and continue to be on yo-yo diets. You need to determine how much protein, carbohydrate and fat you're eating. Your body needs these, but in the right amounts. What your body doesn't need are the saturated fats you find in all the processed foods, fatty meats and whole milk and cheeses. It's important that you realize that milk, cheese and meat aren't bad for you, it's the saturated fat in them which are bad. So learn to trim off the fat, change your milk to 1% or skim. Eat less cheese or cheese with less saturated fat. Mozzarella has less saturated fat that most others, but this doesn't mean you can smother your food with it either.

Avoid the snacking (I call this grazing) that only adds calories and problems. Very few of us are drying from starvation when we head for mid-morning, mid-afternoon, late-evening snacks. How did our parents and grandparents ever survive? I guess they just had to eat apples, oranges, pears and other healthier foods. Another thing to avoid are all the carbonated beverages. I'm not saying they should be eliminated completely. There's a time and a place for these, but how many times a day do you need a "pop." For kids in school it seems to be often. So often in fact that many of them don't even have the lunch money sent with them for "lunch." Instead they blow the money on pop and candy.

If we have pop and candy machines in school because children "want" them, then we should have beer and cigarette machines also because many of them "want" them. If that argument doesn't hold water for beer and cigarettes, then it doesn't hold water for pop and candy either. A "want" is a "want," and a "want" is different than a "NEED." I would also argue that if they weren't snacking on pop and candy, they might be more inclined to eat the foods served rather than waste them. Then we can address the issue about school lunch menus which have way too much fat in them for what the kids need. Since we are responsible for what our children learn and what they eat, it's time we behave like it. As I mentioned earlier, over 25 million girls and boys have high cholesterol problems with even more being overweight, having diabetes or high blood pressure. If this isn't a wake-up call, I don't know what is.

Another problem revolves around our busy work schedules. It might be time to ask ourselves if it's worth it. Most of the people I know who have gone to Europe notice several things: first, they are more relaxed; second, they have longer lunch breaks; and third, they take summer vacations which are several weeks long. We spend so much time competing in this rat race and worrying about who might be getting ahead of us, that we haven't noticed we're killing ourselves and our families. One of the consequences has been eating whatever we can find after we get home, going out to eat, and eating so late that everything we do eat (even if it is good) gets turned into fat as we sleep.

To reduce some of these problems, I offer the following suggestions. Prepare foods in advance. This can be done on the weekend or whenever you get the opportunity. The food can be put in the refrigerator or freezer and used throughout the week when needed. Secondly, think of foods that you can prepare quickly like pastas, fruits, et cetera. Finally, is the issue of eating out. You wouldn't dream of going into a store looking for a television and having someone tell you that you would rather have a car stereo and handing it to you and to pay the cashier on the way out. Yet so many people are used to going and ordering whatever they can find and eating it whether it's any good for them or not.

The same problems existed just a few years ago for non-smokers who went into restaurants and were forced to sit where other people were smoking. Most people I knew would just sit down, annoyed with the smoke, but eat whatever they could find and endure the entire episode. It wasn't until people understood the dangers and risks associated with this and decided they were going to do something about it that things changed. The same problem existed in hospitals. I would walk by the nurses room or respiratory therapy and even doctors lounges and smoke would fill the air. Everyone knew it was unhealthy, but what could you do about it. The answer was simpler than people thought. Once enough people started to stand up and say enough is enough, the system changed. First non-smokers could eat where they could partially breath (although the second-hand smoke was still a problem) and then the area where smokers could smoke was changed for the benefit of all.

The same thing is true about the food we eat in restaurants. Restaurants are supposed to have some of the best chefs available. When you spend your money, they should serve you what you want, not what they want. I encourage people to try different foods and to ask for changes. For example, if something is served in a white sauce (which usually means cream, heavy milk) ask to have the food prepared differently. A creative chef can prepare a food in many different ways. Another suggestion is to ask how many calories, and how much saturated fat is present in a food. Any recipe with a heart next to it should have this information readily available. If they don't know what's in it, how can they claim or suggest that it is heart healthy. Not all foods with a heart next to it are that healthy. In fact, many of the foods without the heart are healthier. In the end, it is the consumer and not the food industry which will determine how healthy the food is. After all, it was the consumer and no one else who recognized the risk of cigarettes. The government and everyone else only jumped on the band wagon after the momentum to make change had started. If you want healthier foods, you have to demand healthier foods. It is after all your health and your money.

Chapter Thirteen.
Concluding Thoughts.

The role of any good physician (in my opinion) is to take care of his/her patients and to help educate them with the idea that they and their family will benefit as a result. Some of us have had the opportunity to study and try to better understand heart disease, what causes it and what we can do about it. During my 23 years with the American Heart Association and the last 13 years researching heart disease, I have been blessed with the opportunity to investigate the reversibility and stabilization of heart disease as a result of my particular training as a Preventive and Nuclear Cardiologist.

The first book *How to Bypass Your Bypass* was written at the request of my friends, family members and patients who were particularly concerned about their risk of heart disease and those they care about. It was tempting (particularly when friends were writing similar books) to write a book early on, in an effort to be one of the first, but I waited more than 10 years before writing my first book. I'm glad I did because much of what I know today (based upon our research over the last 13 years), I didn't know then, and neither did anyone else. It is better to write a book based upon solid research than to guess, knowing that you may be changing your life and the lives of your family and friends, based upon what you're reading.

What we have discovered to be true of heart disease is also true for diabetes, cancer, high blood pressure, obesity and even strokes. As I began lecturing throughout the United States, Europe and the Mediterranean on the research behind the book *How to Bypass Your Bypass*, it became even more obvious that something needed to be done to correct the misinformation being spread today by people looking to make a profit on the health problems and concerns of others. It was because of this that I have written this second book, *The Diet Myth: Keeping Your Heart Forever Young.*

Much of what you and I have read and heard is based upon conjecture, mis-information, a "good idea," and just plan nonsense. As I travel around the country to lecture, I find the same questions and confusion. Some of it caused by honest efforts of some individuals to report the newest information before anyone else. Most of it, however, is based on an effort to make money. While I have nothing against people earning a living, and this approach may seem like a good idea to the person making the money, it isn't helping anyone who is looking for and needs the help.

There may even be some people who think what they're doing is helping others. Many of them are not only fooling you, they're fooling themselves. The purpose of this book isn't to make money. If it does that's fine, but if it helps you and you give it to someone else and it helps them, that's even better. One of the book signings I had was held close to my home. One of the store employees sent a copy of the book to her brother who is a police officer in a New York precinct. He showed the book to several other officers and, to the best of her knowledge, it is still floating around the precinct. One copy sold!

This series of books represents my desire to teach you just as I would my own patients. While I'm not going to replace your doctor, I hope you will share this information with him/her and together work to improve your health and the health of those you love.

Good Health & Bon Appetite!!!